Children's Food Practices in Families and Institutions

This book brings together recent UK studies into children's experiences and practices around food in a range of contexts, linking these to current policy and practice perspectives. It reveals that food works not only on a material level as sustenance but also on a symbolic level as something that can stand for thoughts, feelings, and relationships. The three broad contexts of schools, families and care (residential homes and foster care) are explored to show the ways in which both children and adults use food. Food is used as a means by which adults care for children and is also something through which adults manage their own feelings and relationships to each other which in turn impact on children's experiences.

The book examines the power of food in our daily lives and the way in which it can be used as a medium by individuals to exert power and resistance, establish collective identities and notions of the self and to express moralities about notions of 'proper' family routines and 'good' and 'healthy' lifestyle choices. It identifies inter-generational and intra-generational differences and commonalities in regard to the uses of and experiences around food across a range of studies conducted with children and young people.

This book was published as a special issue of *Children's Geographies*.

Samantha Punch is a senior lecturer in Sociology in the Department of Applied Social Science at Stirling University. Her research interests include rural livelihoods in China, Vietnam and India, youth transitions and migration in Bolivia, children's sibling relationships and birth order. Her recent publications include *Global Perspectives on Rural Childhood and Youth: Young Rural Lives* (2007), *Get Set for Sociology* (with McIntosh, Edinburgh University Press: 2005) and *Sociology: Making Sense of Society* (with Marsh, Keating, Harden, Pearson: 2009).

Ian McIntosh is a senior lecturer in Sociology in the Department of Applied Social Science at Stirling University. His research interests include attitudes to begging, national identities and belonging. Recent publications include *Get Set for Sociology* (with Punch, Edinburgh University Press: 2005) and *English People in Scotland: an Invisible Minority* (with Robertson and Sim, Edwin Mellen Press: Lampeter: 2008).

Ruth Emond is a part time senior lecturer in Social Work in the Department of Applied Social Science at the University of Stirling. She has conducted research in a range of areas relating to vulnerable children and young people, particularly those in institutional care. She works part time as a social worker and play therapist at The Family Change Project in Perth, Scotland where she supports children and young people who have experienced complex trauma.

Children's Food Practices in Families and Institutions

Edited by
Samantha Punch, Ian McIntosh and Ruth Emond

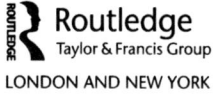

LONDON AND NEW YORK

First published 2011
by Routledge
2 Park Square, Milton Park, Abingdon, Oxon, OX14 4RN

Simultaneously published in the USA and Canada
by Routledge
711 Third Avenue, New York, NY 10017

Routledge is an imprint of the Taylor & Francis Group, an informa business

This book is a reproduction of *Children's Geographies*, vol. 8, issue 3. The Publisher requests to those authors who may be citing this book to state, also, the bibliographical details of the special issue on which the book was based.

Typeset in Times New Roman by Taylor & Francis Books
Printed and bound in Great Britain by TJI Digital, Padstow, Cornwall

British Library Cataloguing in Publication Data
A catalogue record for this book is available from the British Library

ISBN13: 978-0-415-59455-4

Disclaimer
The publisher would like to make readers aware that the chapters in this book are referred to as articles as they had been in the special issue. The publisher accepts responsibility for any inconsistencies that may have arisen in the course of preparing this volume for print.

Contents

1. Introduction   1
   Samantha Punch, Ian McIntosh and Ruth Emond

CHILDREN, FOOD AND INSTITUTIONS

2. Food and its meaning for asylum seeking children
   and young people in foster care
   Ravi K.S. Kohli, Helen Connolly and Andrea Warman   7

3. Children and food practices in residential care:
   ambivalence in the 'institutional' home
   Niku Dorrer, Ian McIntosh, Samantha Punch and Ruth Emond   21

4. Discussant piece: linking, bridging and bonding:
   the importance of a psycho-social perspective for Children
   in Public Care
   Jonathan Stanley   35

CHILDREN, FOOD AND SCHOOLS

5. School lunches: children's services or children's spaces?
   Paul Daniel and Ulla Gustafsson   39

6. 'I don't have to listen to you! You're just a dinner lady!':
   power and resistance at lunchtimes in primary schools
   Jo Pike   49

7. Discussant piece: food and schools
   Ian McIntosh, Ruth Emond and Samantha Punch   63

CONTENTS

CHILDREN, FOOD AND FAMILIES

8. **Children's snacking, children's food: food moralities and family life**
   Penny Curtis, Allison James and Katie Ellis   65

9. **Food and family practices: teenagers, eating and domestic life in differing socio-economic circumstances**
   Kathryn Backett-Milburn, Wendy Wills, Mei-Li Roberts and Julia Lawton   77

10. **Discussant piece: how parenting education and family learning can be set within a tiered intervention framework to aid the development of healthy eating practices**
    Catriona Rioch   89

    Index   92

INTRODUCTION

Food and food practices

Food and food practices lend themselves to sociological and geographical analysis. In particular the study of the relationships that develop around and through food interactions and rituals can bring into focus practices that are often hidden from view; part of an everyday and mundane world frequently so taken for granted that their meaning becomes lost. Research in this growing field brings to light the significance of food and food practices, and the manner in which their study can provide a lens to explore other facets of social life (Jackson 2009a) within a range of different contexts. Food is of course obviously linked to caring, nutrition and the body (Cunningham 2003, Metcalfe *et al.* 2008). The rituals of mealtimes provide scaffolding around which time is organised and through which families and other social groups interact and to a large extent 'do' family. However the significance of the role of food can often be forgotten, partly as a consequence of how fundamental it is, and thus left in the background of sociological analysis. Food practices then are powerful mechanisms of socialisation and can convey a power that can emerge strongly in a range of differing contexts.

Part of taking a 'practices' perspective on food is the view that food works not only on a material level as sustenance but also on a symbolic level as something that can come to stand for thoughts, feelings, and relationships. As a social and symbolic object, food carries and changes meaning with the different uses it can be put to by people in their interactions with each other (McKendrick 2004a, Charon 2007). Part of the objective of studying food practices holistically, within their socio-spatial contexts, is to examine in parallel the ways in which both children and adults use food. Food is not only used as a means by which adults care for children, but it is something through which adults manage their own feelings and relationships to each other which in turn impact on children's experiences. Interactions around food are consequently interpreted from different perspectives and can involve multiple meanings. This is especially the case within contexts such as residential homes where people are brought together from different backgrounds and with very different past experiences (see Dorrer *et al.* this volume).

There has been an increase in research which explores the social significance of food practices in relation to childhood and in interactions between children and adults (Jackson 2009b, James *et al.* 2009a). Recent studies have emphasised the role of food in the demonstration of care and its use for an exchange of affection (e.g. Kaplan 2000, Gillen and Hancock 2006, Punch *et al.* 2009). They have examined how power relationships between adults and children are played out and negotiated via food practices, for example through the contesting of rules for family and school mealtimes (Grieshaber 1997, Alcock 2007, Pike 2008). Such research has demonstrated that food is drawn on as a key tool in the construction of children's identities (James *et al.* 2009a), including the different socio-economic and moral identities of families (Wills *et al.* 2008, James *et al.* 2009b), young people's gendered peer group identities (Valentine 2000), or children's peer group positions within a mixed, multi-ethnic school community (Nukaga 2008). Recent family studies which have explored parents' and children's food practices (e.g. Backett-Milburn *et al.* 2006, Wills *et al.* 2007, James *et al.* 2009b) have also noted the tension between controlling children on the one hand, whilst acknowledging their growing autonomy on the other. Indeed Pike's (2008) analysis of primary school dining rooms illustrates a range of ways in which adults control children's food practices. The authors in this volume continue to develop our understanding of children and food by exploring the themes of space, identity, care, control and power.

Food, space and contexts

This collection began as a set of papers for a one-day conference funded by the Economic and Social Research Council (ESRC) and supported by the Centre for Research on Families and Relationships (CRFR) at the University of Stirling on 11 May 2009. The discussions and debates which followed from this conference enabled this multi-disciplinary edited collection to emerge. Thus the volume builds on recent viewpoints which have appeared in the *Children's Geographies* journal (Cunningham 2003, McKendrick 2004a) by covering three broad contexts, and the related spaces, within which food practices are played out: in care, schools and families.

Over the past two decades the re-consideration of 'space' in analytical approaches to social life, often referred to as a 'spatial turn' (Warf and Arias 2008), has opened up new theoretical perspectives and possibilities. Understanding social life in terms of 'spatiality' calls us to recognise that there is a fundamental interdependence between spaces and ways of being and perceiving (Keith and Pile 1993, Seymour 2007). Our social positions and experiences are shaped in and through specific spaces; and, in turn, spaces are constituted via our ways of interacting with each other and the objects around us. Löw conceptualises space as a 'relational category', as something that 'can be seen as a relational ordering of living entities and social goods' (2008, p. 35).

Conceptualisations of space such as Löw's (2008) definition of the 'duality of space' place emphasis on the continuous construction of social realities through the interlinking of processes of action, structure, and interpretation. Spaces are created in day-to-day activities (through active positioning and being positioned by the actions of others) which produce spatial structures that enable and constrain actions. In the social studies of childhood, work informed by 'spatiality' has demonstrated that in everyday practice boundaries such as those between children's 'local' worlds and wider 'global' influences are blurred and need to be explored in parallel if we are to gain a richer understanding of contemporary childhoods (Holloway and Valentine 2000).

A focus on the way in which different spaces contextualise children's challenges dominant ideas around childhood. For example, Aitken's (2001) analysis of how the separation of the public workplace from the private domestic sphere in the nineteenth century led to transformations in the way children were perceived and how, in turn, this new interpretation of the role of children in society led to the creation of specific moral and regulated spaces as 'proper' places for children. Analyses of children's spaces in the majority or non-Western world, on the other hand, challenge notions of what a 'normal' childhood is (e.g. Punch 2003). 'Spatiality' further permits a view of children as active agents. For example, Christensen *et al.*'s (2000) exploration of children's understandings of time in the family home has highlighted children's negotiation of how space was used for 'own' or shared time. Space and its manipulation, more precisely the movement in and out of the home, played a key role in how the children continuously constructed a sense of belonging and family.

Taken together the studies cited above highlight that the meanings of spaces and practices, as well as the identities constructed within different 'spatialities', are not fixed but marked by simultaneity, juxtaposition, movement, and fluidity in ongoing processes of negotiation. This volume seeks to contribute to these theoretical concerns by considering children's food practices across three different settings: care homes (both foster and residential care), schools and families.

All the authors display a concern with what can be called the symbolic significance of food and food practices. Food can be a powerful medium through which caring and trust can be achieved and reinforced and a sense of belonging created (Kohli *et al.*, Dorrer *et al.*); through which a 'family' and a 'home' can be created and maintained (Dorrer *et al.*, Curtis *et al.*, Backett-Milburn *et al.*); a means by which people, particularly children, can exert a degree of agency and resistance (Pike, Daniel and Gustafsson); and conversely as a means for exerting power and control (Curtis *et al.*, Dorrer *et al.*, Pike). Food and food practices can be a way in which many of these somewhat abstract and intangible concepts and issues are operationalised and made to feel real and have a physical and bodily facticity.

It is our very familiarity with food and the tastes, smells, textures and rituals that are part of our everyday experience of it, that gives it both its significance and ordinariness. The constant presence of food can give it neutrality which can then be harnessed to initiate interactions, relationships and serve as a confirmation of trust, belonging and caring that can be instant and deeply felt – the examples given by Kohli *et al.* of providing young asylum seeking children food from 'home' is clear evidence of this. Closely held, yet vague and difficult to define, notions of the family and the home are in many ways constituted and realised around food. Food is a key way in which family and home life is actually done – as shown most clearly by Dorrer *et al.*, Curtis *et al.* and Backett-Milburn *et al.*. To this end the meal and the ideal of 'eating together' is central (see also McKendrick 2004b).

This volume brings out the ways in which food practices – the eating of it, its preparation and cooking, and the provision of it – are thoroughly infused with morality. This is emphasised in the research by Curtis *et al.* and Daniel and Gustafsson where notions of good and bad are played out via food. In particular food is meshed into contested moralities about appropriate behaviour for young people and children which are clearly class-based in character. As such 'appropriate' food practices are implicated in patterns of resistance and rejection ['strategies of resistance' Pike] and power and compliance. The limits of children's abilities to be fully empowered social actors are often clearly shown around the intricacies of food relationships with adults and can be fought over in relation to eating habits. A moral economy of food is illustrated across the research settings of families, residential care and schools.

The authors here share a similar approach and perspective – and also methodologies – in relation to seeing children and young people as knowledgeable social actors. This is empirically shown within a range of differing contexts which set varying limits to their power and agency and the manner in which food and food practices are implicated in this is brought out. Food can enable some forms of behaviour and curtail others. The differing interactional and institutional contexts – school, classroom, foster care, residential care etc. – are different spaces [or Bourdieu's fields] with particular matrix of rules, regulations and expectations and peculiar micro-culture and histories. This shared approach across the settings gives a good point of comparison for assessing the revelatory nature of studying food and food practices in their different forms and guises and the meanings generated for individuals as they move through these spaces. The need for more research of differing contexts to empirically bring out the specific and commonalities of such spaces and thus add to our general understanding of the role of food practices within the lives of young people and children is also highlighted.

Several common themes emerge from the research contexts presented here. Perhaps most overarching and most exciting is the acknowledgement that the study of food should, and clearly is, moving far beyond merely considering its nutritional importance but toward the study of food as a powerful symbol of relationships, emotions, social structures and behaviours. This volume highlights that we are starting to understand the complexity of food and food related practices. There are a number of themes which emphasise the symbolic nature of food including the use of food as a lens, the shared meaning of food, food as a means of measuring 'success' and food as a means of resistance.

Food as a lens

By considering food as a lens into daily life (Jackson 2009a), researchers are able to illuminate wider issues within a variety of social contexts. The study of food acts as a window into the everyday life of children at home (Backett-Milburn *et al.*, Curtis *et al.*), school (Daniel and Gustafsson, Pike) and care (Dorrer *et al.*, Kohli *et al.*). Whilst each of these studies highlights different aspects of food practices there are some interesting commonalities. For example, the way in which the formal professional systems involved in food in care and in school focuses very much on the nutritional context of food at the expense of the powerful narratives that the children, and indeed the staff, are recounting about the experience and meaning of food. Food practices are also used to create or reinforce hierarchies within families and organisations, such as dinner ladies (Pike), cooks, domestic staff and care staff (Dorrer *et al.*), foster children and birth children (Kohli *et al.*). Power is central to the way in which food was used, accessed and experienced within these studies.

Shared meanings

One of the most striking issues that emerge from the work presented here is the variation in meaning given to food and how important it is that meaning is understood and shared in order for relationships to develop and capital to be established. For example, in Kohli *et al.*'s study the children are able to recognise the giving of food as symbolic of welcome and nurture. Food is a means to belong. By contrast many of the children in the paper by Dorrer *et al.* recount feeling overwhelmed and confused by the giving and sharing of food. Despite staff viewing food as a means of welcoming children this meaning is not shared by the children themselves. Food is therefore often rejected or resisted – perhaps as a means of rejecting the care on offer or also because it is not recognised as such. The importance of shared meanings extends to adult practices. There seems to be confusion and mistrust between adults or adults and professional systems around food. This is starkly illustrated in Pike's research. Children are therefore often moving between different value/belief systems around food even within one social context.

Food as a means of measuring 'success'

Clearly across the research contexts there is a sense that many of the activities that take place around children are not necessarily tangible or measurable – how is 'good parenting' or 'good care' measured or identified? Parents, care staff, dinner ladies, foster carers all seem to be striving to identify for themselves a sense that what they are doing is 'good enough'. Often the 'ideal family' is drawn on in an attempt to do this – in the study by Curtis *et al.* there is a real sense of 'proper families doing proper food'. This extends to the children's home where staff draw on their own family experiences or the abstract 'ideal family' in order to guide food practices, such as sitting around a table (see also McIntosh *et al.* in press).

Far more poignant are the examples of 'good parents' being able to attune to their child's needs. Curtis *et al.* provide the example of the parent who knows that their child needs a snack when he/she comes home from school. This individual flexibility and knowledge of a child is far less demonstrated by those working within the formal systems of care and school.

Food as a means of resistance

Finally, many of the authors highlight the important role that food and food practices can play in the resistance of power and control by adults (Pike) and children (Curtis *et al.*, Dorrer *et al.*). What is striking is how important a shared understanding of the 'rules' of this resistance are in order for them to be both effective and understood. In the work by Dorrer *et al.*, Kohli *et al.* and Pike there is a sense that these children are having to learn and accommodate new rules. What is perhaps seen as playful at home is seen as deviant or challenging in another context (or vice versa). It is not only the formal food practices that children and adults have to learn but also the informal rules and expectations.

Children's food practices

The edited collection highlights the ways in which food can offer us a window into the often private worlds of children. It shows the extent to which previous food practices and meanings that have been instilled in children and adults are carried on into other relationships and social contexts. More needs to be known about this process and about how best it can be managed and explored. Clearly the similarities between the studies are easier to comprehend than the differences; the latter being related mainly to the different settings within which the research was conducted. The main thrust of all the studies is to reveal the power and significance of food and food practices within people's daily lives. Taken together then the research conducted for this volume clearly asserts the power of food in our daily lives and the way in which it can be used as a medium by individuals to exert power and resistance, establish collective identities and notions of the self and to express, often class-based, moralities about notions of 'proper' family routines and 'good' and 'healthy' lifestyle choices and behaviour.

Acknowledgements

We would like to thank the Economic and Social Research Council for funding our research and the final dissemination conference which brought these authors together, ESRC award reference number: RES-000-23-1581.

Samantha Punch, Ian McIntosh and Ruth Emond
Department of Applied Social Science
University of Stirling
Stirling, FK9 4LA
Scotland

References

Aitken, S., 2001. *Geographies of young people. The morally contested spaces of identity*. London: Routledge.
Alcock, S., 2007. Playing with rules around routine: children making mealtimes meaningful and enjoyable. *Early Years*, 27 (3), 281–293.
Backett-Milburn, K., Wills, W., Gregory, S., and Lawton, J., 2006. Making sense of eating, weight and risk in the early teenage years: views and concerns of parents in poorer socio-economic circumstances. *Social Science & Medicine*, 63 (3), 624–635.

Charon, J., 2007. *Symbolic interactionism. An introduction, an interpretation, an integration.* 9th ed. New Jersey: Pearson Prentice Hall.

Christensen, P., James, A., and Jenks, C., 2000. Home and movement: children constructing 'family time'. *In*: S. Holloway and G. Valentine, eds. *Children's geographies: playing, living, learning.* London: Routledge.

Cunningham, C., 2003. A fruitful direction for research in children's geography: fat chance? *Children's Geographies*, 1 (1), 125–127.

Gillen, J. and Hancock, R., 2006. A day in the life: exploring eating events involving two-year-old girls and their families in diverse communities. *Australian Journal of Early Childhood*, 31 (4), 23–29.

Grieshaber, S., 1997. Mealtime rituals: power and resistance in the construction of mealtime rules. *British Journal of Sociology*, 48 (4), 649–666.

Holloway, S. and Valentine, G., 2000. Spatiality and the new studies of childhood. *Sociology*, 34 (4), 763–783.

Jackson, P., 2009a. Introduction: food as a lens on family life. *In*: P. Jackson, ed. *Changing families, changing food.* Basingstoke: Palgrave Macmillan.

Jackson, P., ed., 2009b. *Changing families, changing food.* Basingstoke: Palgrave Macmillan.

James, A., Kjørholt, A.T. and Tingstad, V., eds., 2009a. *Children, food and identity in everyday life.* Basingstoke: Palgrave Macmillan.

James, A., Curtis, P., and Ellis, K., 2009b. Negotiating family, negotiating food: children as family participants?'. *In*: A. James, A.T. Kjørholt and V. Tingstd, eds. *Children, food and identity in everyday life.* Basingstoke: Palgrave Macmillan.

Kaplan, E., 2000. Using food as a metaphor for care: middle-school kids talk about family, school, and class relationships. *Journal of Contemporary Ethnography*, 29 (4), 474–509.

Keith, M. and Pile, S., 1993. *Place and politics of identity.* London: Routledge.

Löw, M., 2008. The constitution of space: the structuration of spaces through the simultaneity of effect and perception. *European Journal of Social Theory*, 11 (1), 25–49.

McIntosh, I., Dorrer, N., Punch, S., and Emond, R., in press. 'I know we can't be a family, but as close as you can get': Displaying families within an institutional context. *In*: E. Dermott and J. Seymour, eds. *Displaying family: new theoretical directions in family and intimate life.* Basingstoke: Palgrave Macmillan.

McKendrick, J., 2004a. The diet of children's geographies. *Children's Geographies*, 2 (2), 287–295.

McKendrick, J., 2004b. Fallacies surrounding the geography of family eating. *Children's Geographies*, 2 (2), 293–295.

Metcalfe, A., Owen, J., Shipton, G., and Dryden, C., 2008. Inside and outside the school lunchbox: themes and reflections. *Children's Geographies*, 6 (4), 403–412.

Nukaga, M., 2008. The underlife of kid's school lunchtime: negotiating ethnic boundaries and identity in food exchange. *Journal of Contemporary Ethnography*, 37 (3), 342–380.

Pike, J., 2008. Foucault, space and primary school dining rooms. *Children's Geographies*, 6 (4), 413–422.

Punch, S., 2003. Childhoods in the majority world: miniature adults or tribal children? *Sociology*, 37 (2), 277–295.

Punch, S., McIntosh, I., Emond, R., and Dorrer, N., 2009. Food and relationships: children's experiences in residential care. *In*: A. James, A.T. Kjørholt and V. Tingstad, eds. *Children, food and identity in everyday life.* Basingstoke: Palgrave Macmillan.

Valentine, G., 2000. Exploring children and young people's narratives of identity. *Geoforum*, (312), 257–267.

Warf, B. and Arias, S., 2008. *The spatial turn: interdisciplinary perspectives.* London: Routledge.

Wills, W., Backett-Milburn, K., Gregory, S., and Lawton, J., 2008. 'If the food looks dodgy I dinnae eat it': teenagers' accounts of food and eating practices in socio-economically disadvantaged families. *Sociological Research Online*, 13 (1–2).

Food and its meaning for asylum seeking children and young people in foster care

Ravi K.S. Kohli,[a] Helen Connolly[a] and Andrea Warman[b]

[a]Department of Applied Social Studies, University of Bedfordshire, Luton, UK; [b]Who Cares Trust, London, UK

There is little in the existing literature in refugee studies, foster care and the anthropology of food about the ways refugee and asylum seeking children regard food. This piece reports on two initiatives that delineate ways children seeking asylum and their carers understand food. The first is a research study examining unaccompanied asylum seeking children's perception of the United Nations Convention on the Rights of the Child, within which they focus on food and survival after arrival in the UK. The second, based on interviews with foster carers, is a practice orientated enquiry about food and its meaning in foster care. The findings suggest that food is related to many aspects of finding sanctuary, negotiating belonging within the foster family, and can powerfully evoke being at 'home' in a new land.

Introduction

At the beginning I did not like the food but now I have no problem. I have even eaten monkey in London, although is too expensive. (Faiges-Hijon 2005, p. 23)

This is the voice of Kalil, a boy of 16 from the Democratic Republic of Congo, who came to the UK as an unaccompanied asylum seeking child and was asked to talk about what being at 'home' meant to him, both in the past and now. He had come far from his homeland in order to be safe, and to belong somewhere and to be successful in his own life with a little help from others (Kohli 2008). Describing the process of adjusting to a new environment, like many of his contemporaries, he looked back, tried to make sense of his present circumstances, and looked forward into the future with a mixture of hope and anxiety. His position within the country of sanctuary was liminal, as it is for many young people seeking asylum. His story of food expresses some of the tensions inherent in the lives of refugee children. It is these stories that we dwell on here, looking at children who have escaped war and famine, through a discourse on food and its meaning to them and their carers. In 2007, of the estimated 31.7 million people of concern to the United Nations High Commission for Refugees, about half were children – some 14 million (UNHCR 2008). Out of these, 3525 children came alone to the UK and made an application for asylum (Home Office 2008), a trickle among the substantial flow of displaced people world wide. At the end of March 2008, 3500 unaccompanied children were being looked after by Social Services Departments in England under s20 of the Children Act 1989 (DCSF 2008), about one in twenty of all looked after children. It is not known how many of them were in foster care.

At present, insights into the ways refugee and asylum seeking children think about and consume food are primarily restricted to the nutritional, with a major focus on destitution and survival (UNHCR 2008). Equally, within the broad arena of the study of foodways and food and culture, while migration and the transplantation of food habits and customs receives diligent appraisal (Herbert 2006, Marte 2007), there is as yet little understanding of what food means to asylum seeking children beyond its face value as a means of survival. Thirdly, within research on foster care there is substantial evidence that the success of placements in families is strongly related to the quality of care that children and young people receive, and more specifically, to carers' abilities to sustain relationships with the children they look after (Sinclair 2005). Yet there is little evidence about the role that food plays in the everyday strategies used by foster carers to establish and continue these relationships. So in the growing body of knowledge about effective foster care for vulnerable children, food is a footnote, rarely a major item of study or concern. Therefore, when standing at the intersection of these three dimensions, food does not appear in any comprehensive way as a sustaining, replenishing, comforting, and sense making aspect of the lives of children seeking asylum. Particularly for those who seek asylum alone and are cared for by foster families within new nations, nothing has yet been traced about the ways in which they negotiate their way to the host table. In effect we know little about their tracks and strategies of stepping up to the plate, so to speak, of doing so not only to ensure their survival, but also to exercise their right to a legitimate space within which they can develop a sense of coming back 'home' through creating their own menu of choices. So, despite the foundations of knowledge within refugee studies, foster care and the anthropology of food (Mintz and Du Bois 2002), we have little understanding of their navigational skills, or the ways they use food as a vector in their calculations of arrival and resettlement into foreign spaces.

Here, we attempt to develop a framework of understanding that children seeking asylum and their foster families can use as they look for safety, belonging and sanctuary within the United Kingdom. We offer some evidence of ways families and the children that they care for co-construct environments that are food friendly, welcoming, and offer a taste of nostalgia and fellowship in what in many instances are hostile social environments and uncertain times. We propose that food, and thinking about food, is full of significance for asylum seeking children as a way of sustaining the shoots of recovery and re-growth, because it symbolises the surrender and recapture of the smell, taste and texture of ordinary life, whether it is 'strange' and comes in a Styrofoam container, or whether it is part of a balanced plateful of evocative goodness. We report on two initiatives that have developed in parallel. The first is a research study undertaken by one of us (Helen) to understand asylum seeking children's perception of the United Nations Convention on the Rights of the Child, where they talk of the perils and pitfalls of receiving care, and of their fortitude and tenacity in making sense of their circumstances. Here, they evoke some important metaphors related to food, survival, and accomplishment. The second is a practice orientated initiative coordinated by one of us (Andrea) with foster carers who give accounts of the meaning of food within their households, and the strategies they use to ensure that children feel welcomed and understood through foods that affirm hope, order and solidarity in their lives. Our preliminary exposition highlights the need to think about food in foster care as a significant aspect of linking, bridging and bonding with asylum seeking children as they establish their entitlements to being found after feeling lost in their journeys to 'home'.

Food and survival

> They just ask for food. 'Give us a goat to eat' they say. So we just give them one.(Turton 2004, p. 28)

The currency of food and its association with power are highlighted by Turton's (2004) vignette in interviewing the Mursi people in Ethiopia. Caught between raiders of different sorts who took without asking, their flimsy hold on their own possessions and livelihoods illuminates above the uneven ways in which food distribution occurs. It is generally a fact of war that food becomes scarce, and that people displaced during times of war, meet famine or at least threats to being able to reliably find food in sufficient quantities to sustain life (UNHCR 2002). Moreover, famine is not just one of the consequences of war, but a tool of aggression that shreds civic structures and rhythms, making life that was perhaps once smooth into a raw and sharp existence (McRae and Zwi 2007). Witnessing the ways war kills ways of life, Summerfield illustrates the survival of Guatemalan Mayans through persecution in the 1980s. He observes that,

> Survivors feel that their collective body has been wounded, one which includes the ants, trees, domestic animals, and ancestors gathered across generations. To them the burning of crops by the army was an attack not just on their food sources but on the symbol which most fully represented them as the people of maize – it was genocide. (Summerfield 2000, p. 233)

Wars as well as natural disasters raise the issue of food insecurity, where aid agencies deal in complex humanitarian emergencies, outlining logistical difficulties, threats, vulnerabilities and costs (FAO 2008). Following the precept first articulated by Sen (1981), Turton (2003) notes that those who starve in a famine do so not because there is insufficient food available but because they have insufficient *entitlement* to food – making the nutritional aspects of food a clearly demarked political issue, not just an economic one. Here, those who are powerful are able to use food to maintain their place and position while simultaneously distancing themselves from those less powerful. In this context, food is a divider, not a connector and one within which children who become refugees are said to be particularly vulnerable, moving away from places and people who have reliably cared for them and protected them (UNHCR 1994). Many remain displaced within their countries of origin, or perhaps make it to a refugee camp across one national border. The machinery of humanitarian assistance swings into action (Hofman *et al.* 2004), aiming though selective feeding programmes and increased healthcare to save lives, reduce and prevent further malnutrition, and protect livelihoods (Shoham 2004). The definitive guidelines issued by UNHCR on the protection and care of refugee children (1994) note that the single most important factor in predisposing refugee children to high mortality rates during the emergency phase is an inadequate food ration. In the seemingly neutral language of this United Nations agency, the primary focus within emergency situations is on quantity and type of intake of food and water, with questions of culturally or socially permissible foods, and questions of choice, receiving less attention.

Yet as with famine and food, the issue of power never quite goes away in the relationships between those in need of food and their helpers. Food parcels, in themselves manifestations of entitlement distributed in systematic ways to those in priority need, come to symbolise the receipt of gifts from donors. Moreover, as Harrell-Bond *et al.* (1992) forcefully argue, the relationship between refugees and humanitarian agencies is run along thin lines of moral order where control by donors and gratitude by supplicants becomes a standard feature of using food for survival. For the majority of people who are refugees, the possibility of using the food they are given to barter and exchange for other goods, or to vary their diets, exists only in the shadows. In the light of ordinary days as receivers of charity, food determined by the donor is what you get, and their only reciprocal gift beyond gratitude, is compliance.

In all instances therefore, when faced with danger from enemies or gifts from helpers, the issue of how food is controlled shows itself in a variety of ways, through a process of persistent negotiation with powerful players. For most refugees in the world, being still and learning to regulate the rules that govern survival become essential components of day to day life. Very few refugee children move far away from the arenas of conflict. They and their families cannot afford to. They live and die where circumstances have taken them, within the limited choices that are available to them. Sometimes however, some children move far from their homelands, because their families have the resources to get them false papers, to pay for agents, or because they have some connection with the country they are aiming for (Robinson and Segrott 2002). It is to these extended journeys that we now turn, where issues of food echo matters of survival, yet also move into matters of choice and the refurbishment of living.

Food and asylum

Then there was food. All these burgers, cherry cokes, hot dogs, grilled cheese sandwiches, apple pies à la mode, and dozens of different candy bars that had to be sampled... Fast food has the advantage of being portable... It is a perfect invention for someone hungry all the time, as I was. (Simic 1998, p. 127)

This evocation distils one sense of coming to a new land as a refugee child, where the journey opens out new food possibilities, with the temptation to snack, to be quick, and to keep on the move, grazing whimsically. Perhaps ironically, Simic (1998) also contrasts the above with the slow and sedentary food of his homeland, eaten while sitting at the table. In the sugar rush of arrival, the new carbohydrate and calorie rich world appears to displace the older habits and customs. Yet after arrival, what does food mean to refugee children beyond the excitement of a host country full of supermarkets, takeaway outlets, sweetshops and restaurants? The picture is mixed.

It is now relatively clear that those who manage to come to the doorstep of the richest nations may sometimes arrive with health difficulties related to insufficiency of food, as well as psychosocial difficulties expressed through their relationship with food. For example, Sellen *et al.* (2002) observe that among refugee children who come to the UK to seek asylum, there is a high prevalence of poor diets and limited access to food, particularly in the first two years after arrival. Von Folsach and Montgomery (2006), in a review of literature related to several asylum seeking children in Sweden, identify Pervasive Refusal Syndrome among them, with a main clinical feature being food refusal, lethargy and fatigue, allied to a collapse in their abilities to look after themselves or interact with others. These bleak pictures are at times reinforced and ameliorated by the contexts within which the children are placed. Faiges-Hijon (2005) names a persistent sense of dislocation associated with food, with almost all young people in her research describing food in their locality as unhealthy, not fresh, prepared in a hurry, and marketed in unfamiliar ways. They also noted how alien their own tastes felt, for monkey or crocodile meat, and how expensive food that was cheap at home was in the UK in comparison. Stanley's (2001) survey of young separated refugees in the UK considers the importance of being in places where 'home' food was accessible. It points out that having little money, poor cooking facilities and rudimentary skills in preparing food, lead some of them to feel isolated, and others to making a choice between buying food *or* clothes from their restricted allowances, but not both. Going hungry, for them, reinforced how dependant they were on the kindness and will of others to provide food for them – as if the gift recreated those primal experiences of being supplicants as refugees – and as a consequence how close they remained to dislocation.

When outlining some of the contributions foster carers make to these young people's lives, Wade *et al.* (2005) and Chase *et al.* (2008) refer in their research to the importance of food for asylum seeking children in the UK, allowing a brief glimpse of complex exchanges that we dwell on in detail below. For example, Wade *et al.* (2005) note in their study of how social services respond to the needs of unaccompanied minors that in many cases, advice about nutrition and help with domestic skills formed part of the core work undertaken by carers and support workers. Young people often needed assistance to familiarise themselves with shopping, with the safe use of cooking appliances, to develop their cooking skills and to identify places where foodstuffs familiar to them could be obtained. Chase *et al.* (2008) trace the emotional well being of 54 young people seeking asylum in the UK. Sixty percent of them had experienced foster care at some point in their resettlement journey. Not all foster care was experienced as good. As with indigenous children, aspects of ambivalence with no clear feelings of belonging or safety, and being seen as a child in transition, or as a cipher for monetary gain, occluded their experiences and heightened tensions in the foster home. However, among the gloom, they also confirm that where foster care worked well for these children, it was characterised by places that offered emotional support, stability, love, affection, a mother and/or father figure, clear rules and guidance, and plenty of good food.

Within the limits of the existing literature, perhaps it is no surprise that where food and borders exist, so do issues of entitlement and belonging among the vagaries of resettlement. Hunger and eating enough, longing and wanting 'home' food, the capacity to be in charge of one's health and well being through eating well, and dependence on the kindness of strangers, all make cameo appearances in recent research in the UK. It is these aspects that we now examine further.

The HEAR ME (Hearing Experiences of Asylum and Resettlement) study

In the HEAR ME study 30 unaccompanied asylum seeking young people aged between 12 and 21 discussed their asylum and resettlement experiences in the United Kingdom and how they thought these compared with the international standards contained within the United Nations Convention on the Rights of the Child 1989. They were accessed via social workers in four Children's Services Departments in England from a broad sample of young asylum seekers in care. Following Eastmond's (2007) framework of understanding narratives in forced migration research, each young person was encouraged to tell their story of departure, arrival, and day to day life in the UK, often from positions of liminality, with a strong emphasis on hearing their heartfelt accounts in sympathetic and respectful ways. While each conversation with a young person was taped, ensuring confidentiality and working at a pace of story-gathering that allowed privacy and reassurance to be maintained became key aspects of engagement over time. The process of data collection was iterative, with several meetings with each young person. Initial engagements focussed on building trust and companionship, with subsequent encounters allowing the young person to reflect on, among other aspects of resettlement, their experiences of food. All tapes were transcribed, and data analysed using qualitative data analysis software. The observations on food were organised into the themes presented below.

The demographic characteristics of the participants reflected the current and broader pattern for refugee and asylum seeking children arriving in the United Kingdom. A large number of the participants had arrived from Afghanistan but also from other countries where conflict and disorder have long prevailed. These included particular conflict zones in the Middle East, the Eastern Horn of Africa and West and Southern Africa. The majority had experienced long journeys brokered by agents, a few had been trafficked and others had been brought to the country under private fostering arrangements. In order to preserve anonymity, each young person was asked to choose an alternative name for themselves. These alternatives are used here.

A key observation has been that food details and food experiences often appeared in the young people's plots, thoughts and evaluations. Moreover, while these experiences featured regularly throughout the participants' reflections on a number of the UNCRC standards, they were potently narrated in relation to their foster care experiences. Furthermore, they were also central to how young people made sense of whether Article 20 of the UNCRC framework had been sufficiently engaged in this care setting. This Article sets standards for all children in substitute care. It states that children who move out or cannot remain in their environments of origin should be entitled to *special protection and assistance* by State Parties and that alternative care should be made available to them, including foster care. While the UNCRC imposes this duty it does not specify what special protection and assistance means. Yet, if the whole UNCRC framework works as the scaffolding within which the lives of children can safely grow, it has to be appreciated in its fullness and understood and delivered as a series of articulated bridges between the various Articles it contains (Kohli and Connolly 2008). As such, the standards for safeguarding and supporting children in foster care also form natural links with other articles of the UNCRC. These are apparent in provisions such as those relating physical survival and healthy development (Article 6) and a sufficient standard of living that includes adequate nutrition, clothing and housing conditions (Article 27); the right to physical and psychological recovery (Article 39); freedom to actively appreciate their own culture, religion and language (Article 30) and the right to enjoy leisure and cultural pursuits (Article 32); and the rights to participation, where children should influence the decisions that shape the forms, movement and tempo of their lives (Article 12).

In the stories they told, the interplay of these life-enabling rights in the UNCRC were recognised by the young participants of the HEAR ME study as central to the creation of a care environment that clarified the foggy conditions of Article 20. It also offered them a sense of sanctuary, reprieve and 'home'. Their appreciation of the permeable and fluid nature of the Convention, and the influence of other Articles on foster care was shown in their conversations around food. Indeed, by prioritising food throughout their discussions on rights, young people produced narratives that confirmed the centrality of food as a means of linking and bridging across key Articles in the UNCRC framework. We now direct our focus towards the finer details of their discourse.

Food as the first refuge

We begin by looking at the point preceding the imbroglio of the sugar rush. While the literature on the lives and circumstances of refugees tells us a little of their circumstances before leaving and of their journeys to sanctuary towards the world's richest nations, it is well furnished with accounts of young people's arrival, suggesting that they often alight on new shores tired, confused, famished and fearful of what lies beyond (Ayotte 2000). Kohli (2007) and Hopkins and Hill (2008) confirm, through closely observed narratives of unaccompanied minors in England and Scotland, that food, in such contexts of uncertainty and flux, provides a practical and psychological fix that allowed them to find their bearings. Similarly, in this study, food as a means of evoking past experiences echoed throughout the accounts offered by the young participants. Arrival stories referred to their encounters with border control, to entry into the care system, and for many, being introduced to a foster family. Food appeared central in young people's memories of when they were first introduced to their foster families, and some recounted tales of food as being the first refuge. This is encapsulated in the comments by two young people offered below.

> Social services was contacted that night and all I remember was I was still locked in a cell and the police officer came to say that she had good news for me that I was going to go to a house, have good nights sleep, a good shower and some good food. I was picked up from the police station by social services who had arranged for me to go to a foster house where I was looked after for a couple of months. (Aura from Uganda)

> Then they took us to a foster home and we had our first meal in the UK. (Abdat from Eritrea)

In these early stages of arrival, food therefore had the capacity to function as one of the first signs of the hospitality and security that lay ahead. In this respect, the level of care that was represented in this first meal had the power to communicate how young people felt safe after arrival or how they began to invest hope in being found and reclaimed.

Feeling found and reclaimed

For many young people, their food experiences in foster care were at the heart of whether their hopes turned into reality. For those who spoke of being found and reclaimed, there was often a consolatory logic to the words they used to tell their stories, and to make sense of their lives as those stories were told. There was sadness about their losses and bereavements. This was offset by the light and reparative tone that filled their accounts of settings they experienced as warm and carers they experienced as willing to nurture. Feeling food secure, being cooked for, sharing the table, participating in house menus and food shopping were all part of the light and reparation and of young people feeling consoled by the process of beginning to belong again. One of the participants enlivens this enabling function of food:

> Food is about compassion. I left home and I left my parents to come here. Food is the thing that makes me feel security and like there is more love for me. I feel secure and protected here. I feel like when I am there I am at my fathers home and she (the foster carer) gives me love the way that my mother used to give me love and I feel good in this love. (Grace, from the Democratic Republic of Congo)

Reinforced displacement

However, just as food can act as a catalyst in the enabling process, a significant number of young people spoke about power and food and the ways it could be used to push them away from a sense of safety and belonging (see also Dorrer *et al.* this volume). In these instances, foster carers were reported to have exercised control over food in ways that not only prohibited the successful integration in the home but that also reinforced young people's broader feelings of displacement. The comments below from Ayesha from Afghanistan distil this:

> In the foster carer's home it was like in prison. She had a shop and all day she was in her shop and I was alone at home and it was a nightmare for me. It was a new country and I expected different. It was my dream to come to Europe and I lost all my family in a war and I thought Europe was a very good place in my thoughts but actually it was different. She worked from morning until evening and she cooked once a day... I wasn't full and I didn't have enough food, has anyone else said they didn't have enough food? It is not your home and you just have to wait for that piece of chicken and for the person who just come it make you more sad. I used to cry a lot and not come out of my room.

Morsels of freedom

While the above story and other similar stories raise some concerns around the issue of food security for refugee and asylum seeking children in foster care, it also epitomises the idea of food availability and choice being linked to freedom. This sentiment replicates the bi-dimensional understanding of hunger espoused by American anthropologist Nancy Scheper-Hughes. In work that explored the relationship between hunger and emotion amongst Brazilian women living on the margins, she captured the association between the physical yearning of the belly and the psychosocial consequences of not having food choice (Scheper-Hughes 1992). For them, desirable food remained always out of reach. This phenomenon also found vivid expression in the lives of young people in this study, where they expressed a longing not only for more food but also to a wider variety of food in foster care.

> My social worker told my foster carer that she is supposed to buy fruit and sweets and chocolates for after dinner or anytime that we want and to change the food as well. (Ayesha, from Afghanistan)

She never used to ask me what I would like to eat. She would just buy cheap things from Lidl's and then give it to us to eat. She never bought anything once. Okay, the first Christmas I was there, she went shopping and we went to Sainsbury's and she asked me to pick up an item that I liked and it was like one pound and she had done a whole trolley for her family shopping and she asked me to pick up one thing and that is the only thing she asked me to. You are not supposed to just buy for your own family and then buy cheap stuff for me on the side and just let me eat when you cook. (Georgina, from Nigeria)

In these unkind contexts, young people found themselves reading between the menu, in the sense that they had to understand the text and subtext of what was on offer from the foster carer. In all, food became a symbol for their lowly position and the misuse of power within the foster care household. This lead some to question their own worth, the rules of engagement about food consumption and the reasons for being put on the margin while others were allowed easier access to the dinner table. In some instances, young people reported that they were made to eat separately from adults in the household. They were transfixed to an eating rota in contexts where adults were allowed to graze and roam. They said they could not import or cook foods from their homelands. In a minority of cases, food cooked at the weekend was eaten cold until midweek. This confirmed a strong and lasting sense of food insecurity within households in ways that could not meet their need for the warmth of communal contact. Over time, some of them came to believe that their presence in their foster care setting was not so much about their care, but about the foster carer using them to earn money.

Overall, the young people's stories referred to the interdependence between safety and belonging and power in relation to food within foster care. Yet the study in its design did not elicit the views of foster carers themselves. It is this second dimension that we examine now via a separate enquiry, where foster carers were engaged in giving their perspectives about food. By doing so, we link the lived reality for unaccompanied children to the good that could happen in foster care if circumstances focussed more clearly on optimistic engagements with them.

Food and integration: the 'Recipes for Fostering' initiative

In 2007 the British Association for Adoption and Fostering conducted a small practitioner-led research study within the UK that highlighted ways foster carers welcomed children into their homes. In part, the study identified the importance to foster carers of shopping, cooking and eating together with the children in their care (BAAF 2007). From this an opportunity to explore these issues further when the UK's largest independent fostering agency, Foster Care Associates, provided funding for a new BAAF practice orientated initiative focussing on food in foster care. Ten foster care households involving a total of 12 foster carers were individually approached to contribute to the initiative. These households formed a heterogeneous group, with a mix of local authority and independent fostering providers. They were located in different parts of England, in urban and rural settings. The carers had different kinds and length of fostering experience and they came from diverse ethnic and cultural backgrounds. Some were couples and others were single foster carers. What they shared was a reputation within their nominating agencies of being effective, responsible carers. All the carers were interviewed and their narratives were taped, transcribed, and analysed to identify their perceptions of effective practices in relation to food and foster care. Within a framework of delineating such 'good practice', the initiative explored the part food played in their own life histories, and how this had helped to shape and influence their thoughts about food for the children they cared for. Their stories provided accounts of the key role that foster carers can play in helping children and young people to feel safe and at home in very difficult circumstances. These carers, all portraying optimism in different ways, recognised the significance of food and used it in practical, everyday strategies to build and sustain relationships with the children and young people in their care (Warman 2009).

Here we give examples of some of the findings in the enquiry that deepen and amplify the issues raised within the sample of asylum seeking children in the HEAR ME study.

Welcome: food to use when crossing the border into a foster home

There was shared recognition among the carers that in the early stages of a placement it is important to welcome a new member of the household by finding out about what they like to eat, and involving them in choosing meals and shopping for the ingredients. For children for whom choice had been curtailed, where food had been conditional, or when it had been withheld as a method of punishment, having someone ask them about preferences created fragile and respectful entries into the child's inner worlds, where hunger and fear co-existed. Carers who were looking after asylum seeking young people also showed a growing awareness of the importance of respecting boundaries created by traditions different to their own. They did their homework on acceptable foods, and as a consequence changed their own trajectories of food shopping and serving. An African Caribbean carer looking after an Afghani boy seeking asylum explained:

> I was worried when he first came because I knew he is Muslim, and I knew that there are certain dietary needs, but I didn't know much about it. So I found out a bit and then I asked him. And I realised that his meat would have to come from the halal shop. There's a big Asian population around here and it wasn't hard to find a new halal butcher, and that's where I buy my chicken and my mutton now. And I've learned that for cooking it's not any different. You just clean up the meat, season it and use it in the same way you use any other meat. And I do all my meat shopping there now. To the extent that my old butcher's not speaking to me anymore because he's lost a customer!

Food to look back on and food to look forward to

Some of the carers recognised the role that the smells and tastes of food could play in bridging past and present experiences. One of the carers had been a refugee herself, and her history resonated with many of the experiences that she witnessed when trying to understand a young Afghani man placed in her care. She had been born in Kenya within an Indian family that eventually settled in Uganda. In 1972 after Idi Amin came to power, ordinary life came to an abrupt halt, as for many Gujarati families living in Uganda, when all were given 90 days notice to leave the country. As a child, she was smuggled out hiding in a truck, eating nothing and drinking little. Finally, she and her mother and siblings boarded a flight to the UK, with little money and just a few clothes, depending on the kindness of strangers to keep warm in winter weather. The family settled in a small English town. Of those early arrival times, she recalled

> Because we wanted to eat curry and rice, chapattis, [My mother] couldn't do anything because we couldn't buy anything. All we lived on was bread and soup because she couldn't cook a curry or anything like that because in [our town] there was no Asian shop or anything like that, the only place we could have got it was from Birmingham and we didn't even know where Birmingham existed at the time.

Her recollections showed an honest grasp of her bewilderment at a time of crisis. This led her on to stories of integration, of surviving herself, and finally after many years, of arriving psychologically to a place where she could offer something back to children placed with her who were bewildered too. She showed particular sensitivity to the meaning of food that could provide nourishment, but also be used as a gateway to understanding issues of silence and trust (Kohli 2009). Here, cooking a paratha represented a chance to evoke memories of times gone by, and a window and door appeared in the enclosure of silence that many young asylum seekers live within. She said:

> At the beginning he was very, very quiet, and I knew that was because he didn't know who to trust and who not to trust. Then one morning I was cooking paratha. And he quickly came out of the bathroom. Came quickly downstairs and said, the smell, the smell... My mum used to cook paratha and the smell used to come just like that. And I said, would you like some? And he said, oh yes... Stood there watching me make the paratha, and said, that reminds me of my mum. And I could see tears coming in his eyes as he watched me. So I gave him tea and a paratha and said, tell me about it. Tell me what your mum used to do. And then he began to talk. About his mum, about home. And later about his journey. And he began to trust me. Then he could talk about all the bad things. The things that had happened on his journey here that had been kept locked inside.

This ability to listen, reflect and unlock the meaning of food beyond meeting physical needs was also illustrated by another of the carers, who had learned a great deal from the young man in her care. She was not only now buying and cooking with halal meat, but had also come to understand the reasons for fasting and the kinds of food that he liked to eat to break the fast. She had adapted her own Caribbean dishes to suit his tastes, so that within her home there was a constellation of dishes from across the world, negotiating her history and food preferences with those of the young man she cared for. In this sense, the borders around food were lessened and made more permeable, creating in some ways a novel representation of fusion food.

> Well, he likes my rice and peas, and he'll eat that with a curry made with halal mutton. Or sometimes he likes it with fish – either battered fish from the chip shop, or my fish that I fry up with Jamaican spices. I mix it all up now!

Food, fellowship, and the future

Despite the stories told by young people in the first study, the carers in this enquiry did not describe their territories as mini nation states, with borders, with checks for authenticity of claims, or with acts of defence, mean mindedness and insistence on doing things 'their way'. They did not get the young people to integrate on terms determined by a poor use of power. They understood in a heartfelt way that the young people should not be humbled when coming home to them, but rather that they should have a chance to unfurl their bundled lives and understand that they were in a safe place, a place of opportunity and goodness. They confirmed that boundaries of civility and self respect were needed in order to create a sustainable rhythm of living, but these did not translate into a set of unassailable rules. One foster carer noted that at his table there was an abundance of food from which children could choose whatever they liked. But once it was on their plate, they were responsible for eating everything they had chosen. The simple precept was that choice and responsibility were necessarily part of recreating mealtimes as democratic occasions, with rights to vote allied to being accountable in some way for not wasting food. These rules were embedded with other rules for eating at set times, eating sociably together at the table, identifying favourite things that could punctuate and accentuate a pattern of living – a 'roast dinner' on a Sunday, for example – highlighting a cluster of ways that unpredictable and risk filled lives could rediscover some sense of order. In time, layers of mutual understanding emerged within these fostering households, allowing the children within them to develop interest and ambition in relation to food. In one family, two of the foster carers took great care to teach the young man they looked after to work with them on their allotment, where they grew fruits and vegetables, and helped him to harvest these and bring them home. They taught him to cook, and turned his growing talent in cooking into a livelier prospect of becoming a chef. For a troubled boy, they created a chance to reclaim a sustainable future through eating, cooking, growing food and experimenting with recipes.

While these strategies of generating belonging and success were woven into many of these foster families' stories, they also thought about food legacies – that is, foods that came to symbolise moorings in troubled waters that the children looked back on long after they had left the foster home to lead independent lives. These carers understood the need for continuity of relationships and rituals, as exemplified by one of them and the story of 'The Review Cake'. This foster carer had over 20 years experience and had looked after many young people.

> There was one cake I always liked to make whenever we had a review here. Those meetings could be the most fraught because of course everyone would be here talking about them. And I wanted to try to make everyone feel comfortable in that situation, to feel at ease. I preferred to make my own cake then, rather than just open a packet of shop-bought biscuits. It came out so often over the years that it came to be known as review cake. But my first lot of teenagers called it Hippy Cake. Because it was home made and I used organic ingredients before it was really fashionable to do that. I became famous for that cake! And all of the kids who lived here do all remember it, laugh about it – even now years later when we all get together.

This shared history was being passed on to the next generation when the adults whom she once fostered visited her home bringing their own children.

> I'm meeting their sons and daughters now and they're eating my Hippy Cake! You can use the same mixture and put it in bun cases and the little ones love helping to do that. So we're passing those traditions on along with all of the memories.

Overall, the stories of food and home within the enquiry highlight a number of important features in foster care. Firstly, that children entering a foster carer's home are sensitised to whether there is enough food, and how it is used to create a sense of warmth and welcome. The carers confirmed that food can be used to make sense of one's circumstances and to create sustainable patterns of living. It can integrate fragments from the past, and through evocative acts, offer access to memories that can then reclaim ordinary life after periods of turbulence. Finally, it can generate a sense of skilled living as interests, talents and traditions combine, not through accident, but in using power well and learning and refreshing the rules of ordered and organic lives.

Conclusions

For children seeking asylum, the stakes are high. Their liminal positions reinforce their sensitivity to the presence of powerful adults who have it in their gift to replenish their lives or to harm them. In these volatile contexts food has a central role to play, confirming both their entitlement to protection and care, and also their fragile dependence on others. The stories described in these separate projects give a partial insight to their food journeys, and how these are in constant states of negotiation and flux. From the perspectives of the young people stories emerge that are candid and clear. Food helps them to survive, to feel comforted and enlivened, in ways that engage many of the life giving provisions of the UNCRC. Yet their circumstances also confirm the deep conditionality of giving and taking food in foster care, within a realisation that the boldly stated rights within the UNCRC can only be fully exercised in contexts that are welcoming. Otherwise the young people get by on making the best of diminished resources and circumstances. Where foster carers show a detailed commitment to their well being and use their powers to be kind – in effect bringing them home as citizens of the territories that they govern – asylum seeking children can feel a sustained sense of being replenished through foods of choice. Some of these are foods of longing and familiarity, some are new, and some a combination of the past and present. The foster carers in this research show a capacity to think well beyond nutritional needs, moving in the direction of sustainability and integration. In looking back at the results within these projects, we acknowledge that this work offers a foundation for exploring the ways that food and its multiple meanings are understood for the benefit of children seeking asylum. In our view, it illustrates the need to construct a single project within which the views of children and their carers are gleaned together, rather than as single parallel strands as reported here.

References

Ayotte, W., 2000. *Separated children coming to Western Europe. Why they travel and how they arrive*. London: Save the Children.

British Association of Adoption and Fostering, 2007. *Who am I and what do I do?* London: BAAF.

Chase, E., Knight, A., and Statham, J., 2008. *The emotional well-being of young people seeking asylum in the UK*. London: British Association of Social Workers.

Department for Children, Schools and Families (DCSF), 2008. *Children looked after in England (including adoption and care leavers) year ending 31 March 2008* [online]. Available from: http://www.dcsf.gov.uk/rsgateway/DB/SFR/s000810/SFR23-2008_Final.pdf [Accessed 9.4.2009].

Eastmond, M., 2007. Stories as lived experience: narratives in forced migration research. *Journal of Refugee Studies*, 20 (2), 248–264.

Faiges-Hijon, A., 2005. *The concept and recreation of home amongst unaccompanied asylum seeking and refugee young people in Britain* [online]. 3rd Annual Forced Migration Student. Conference, Oxford Brookes University, Oxford / UK, 13–14 May 2005. http://www.brookes.ac.uk/schools/planning/dfm/FMSC/P&A/faiges.pdf (accessed 9.4.2009).

FAO, 2008. *The state of food insecurity in the world, 2008*. Rome: Food and Agriculture Organization of the United Nations.

Harrell-Bond, B., Voutira, E., and Leopold, M., 1992. Counting the refugees: gifts, givers, patrons and clients. *Journal of Refugee Studies*, 5 (3/4), 205–225.

Herbert, J., 2006. Migration, memory and metaphor: life stories of south Asians in Leicester. *In*: K. Burrell and P. Panayi, eds. *Histories and memories. Migrants and their histories in Britain*. London and New York: Tauris Academic Studies.

Hofman, C.A., Roberts, L., Shoham, J., and Harvey, P., 2004. *Measuring the impact of humanitarian aid. A review of current practice*. [online]. London: Humanitarian Policy Group at the Overseas Development Institute. Available from: http://www.odi.org.uk/resources/download/237.pdf (Accessed 9.4.2009).

Home Office, 2008. *Asylum Statistics United Kingdom 2007* [online]. Home Office statistical bulletin 21st August 2008. Available from: http://www.homeoffice.gov.uk/rds/pdfs08/hosb1108.pdf (Accessed 9.4.2009).

Hopkins, P. and Hill, M., 2008. Pre-flight experiences and migration stories: the accounts of unaccompanied asylum-seeking children. *Children's Geographies*, 6 (3), 257–268.

Kohli, R.K.S., 2007. *Social work with unaccompanied asylum seeking children*. Palgrave: Macmillan.

Kohli, R.K.S., 2009. Understanding silences and secrets when working with unaccompanied asylum-seeking children. *In*: N. Thomas, ed. *Children, politics and communication. Participation at the margins*. Bristol: The Policy Press.

Kohli, R.K.S. and Connolly, H., 2008. *Fostering children and young people seeking asylum* [online]. Research digest for Community Care Inform. Available from http://www.ccinform.co.uk/ (Accessed 9.4.2009).

Marte, L., 2007. Foodmaps: tracing boundaries of 'home' through food relations. *Food & Foodways*, 15, 261–289.

McRae, J. and Zwi, A.B., 2007. Food as an instrument of war in contemporary African famines: a review of the evidence. *Disasters*, 16 (4), 299–321.

Mintz, S.W. and Du Bois, C.M., 2002. The anthropology of food and eating. *Annual Review of Anthropology*, 31, 99–119.

Robinson, V. and Segrott, J., 2002. *Understanding the decision making of asylum seekers*. Finding 172. Research, Development and Statistics Directorate. Home Office.

Scheper-Hughes, N., 1992. *Death without weeping: the violence of everyday life in Brazil*. Berkeley, CA: University of California Press.

Sellen, D.W., Tedstone, A.E., and Frize, J., 2002. Food insecurity among refugee families in East London: results of a pilot assessment. *Public Health Nutrition*, 5 (5), 637–644.

Sen, A., 1981. *Poverty and famines: an essay on entitlement and deprivation*. Oxford: Oxford University Press.

Simic, C., 1998. Refugees. *In*: A. Aciman, ed. *Letters of transit: reflections on exile, identity, language and loss*. New York: New Press.

Sinclair, I., 2005. *Fostering now. Messages from research*. London: Jessica Kingsley.

Shoham, J., 2004. *Review of the role of nutrition and food security information in assessing the impact of humanitarian interventions*. Background Paper. London: Overseas Development Institute.

Stanley, K., 2001. *Cold comfort. Young separated refugees in England*. London: Save the Children.

Summerfield, D., 2000. War and mental health: a brief overview. *British Medical Journal*, 321 (22), 232–235.

Turton, D., ed., 2003. Conceptualising forced migration. *RSC Working Paper 12*. Oxford: Refugees Study Centre, Oxford University.

Turton, D., 2004. *The meaning of place in a world of movement: lessons from long-term field research in southern Ethiopia*. RSC Working Paper 18. Oxford: Refugees Study Centre, Oxford University.

UNHCR, 1994. *Refugee children. Guidelines for protection and care*. Geneva: UNHCR.

UNHCR, 2002. *Meeting the rights and protection needs of refugee children. An independent evaluation of the impact of UNHCR's activities*. Geneva: UNHCR.

UNHCR, 2008. *2007 Global trends: refugees, asylum-seekers, returnees, internally displaced and stateless persons.* Geneva: UNHCR.

Von Folsach, L.L. and Montgomery, E., 2006. Pervasive refusal syndrome among asylum-seeking children. *Clinical Child Psychology and Psychiatry*, 11 (3), 457–473.

Wade, J., Mitchell, F., and Baylis, G., 2005. *Unaccompanied asylum seeking children. The response of social work services.* London: British Association for Adoption and Fostering.

Warman, A., 2009. *Recipes for fostering.* London: British Association for Adoption and Fostering.

Children and food practices in residential care: ambivalence in the 'institutional' home

Nika Dorrer, Ian McIntosh, Samantha Punch and Ruth Emond
Department of Applied Social Science, University of Stirling, Stirling, Scotland

Using an ethnographic approach, we provide an analysis of food practices in residential care to explore the atypical nature of children's homes as a three-fold space that combines characteristics of 'home', 'institution', and 'workplace'. Residential staff invested considerable effort into recreating a 'family-like' home but the practices and ideals they drew on could be interpreted and experienced in different ways. We demonstrate the difficulty of delineating between 'homely', 'institutional', or work oriented practices. While care workers tried to juggle conflicting demands in child-centred ways, the spaces they created could at times be experienced as constraining by the children and as inhibiting a sense of belonging.

Introduction

Our ESRC-funded research explores the micro-level of everyday food practices within residential homes for children. It seeks to demonstrate that the residential home is a three-fold space which combines characteristics of 'home', 'workplace' and 'institution'. Taking a food practices approach, similar to a family practices approach (Seymour 2007), permits a reflection on the interplay between the demands and practicalities of specific situations and the ideals and wider debates that impact on what people do around food and how they interpret it. Locating the analysis on the micro-level of actions further brings into focus the different ways in which staff and children try to exercise control within a complex and multi-governed environment.

Of particular relevance to the present work is Seymour's research (2005, 2007) on family practices in hotels, pubs and boarding houses as it explores the atypical combination of home and workplace in a single location. The everyday routines and practices described by the families in her study reflect the challenges of integrating the simultaneous demands of providing a home, service to the public and realising ideals about a private family life. Seymour shows that 'family' was 'done' (West and Zimmerman 1987, Silva and Smart 1999) in diverse ways with family practices blurring into workplace practices and vice versa. Practices associated with the 'proper' family (see Backett-Milburn *et al.* this volume, Curtis and James this volume), such as the sharing of a meal around the table, were at times appropriated to serve workplace demands, for example, when parents and children performed 'family' for the business by eating together with their guests, while also using such events for the fulfilment of the perceived parental responsibility of equipping children with etiquette and skills.

We argue that a reflection on food practices can provide a critical insight into the complexity of the residential home, as well as the use of food as a medium of care. While the latter has been discussed, in part, elsewhere (Punch *et al.* 2009) here we seek to highlight the ambivalence and conflicts resulting from the simultaneous enactment of family, work and institutional practices around food. Just as Blunt and Edward 'dismantle the dichotomy between homely and unhomely homes' (2006, p. 26) this paper seeks to demonstrate that an unconventional home can be defined in 'homelike' and 'not-home-like' ways and that it is in practice an intersection of 'private' and 'public' spheres.

Methods

Figure 1 outlines the research objectives which guided the methodological approach of this study. In order to gain an insight into the practicalities and social dynamics that surround food at different points in time, and to access the meanings given to them by children and adults, an ethnographic approach was chosen.

The data was gathered during the course of three-month blocks of semi-participant observation in three residential children's homes in Scotland during which one of the authors (Nika) stayed at the homes for between three and six day-long visits per week, including some overnights. Through the prolonged immersion into the homes' daily life it was possible to obtain a detailed documentation of the nature of interactions involved in the distribution, regulation and consumption of food and to gain an understanding of the meanings attributed to the rituals and routines which surrounded these. Data was collected in fieldnotes, overt audio recordings of mealtime interactions, semi-structured interviews and focus groups with the children and members of staff. Nika gradually gained insider status with the homes by joining into such everyday activities as eating, cleaning, relaxing, and chatting with the children and staff. A primary concern was to enable participants to get to know the researcher and test her trustworthiness so that they could co-determine how, when, and what information they were prepared to share for the purpose of the study. The research was informed by guidelines of ethics for researching with children (Alderson and Morrow 2004) and the previous work of Emond (2005) and Punch (2002).

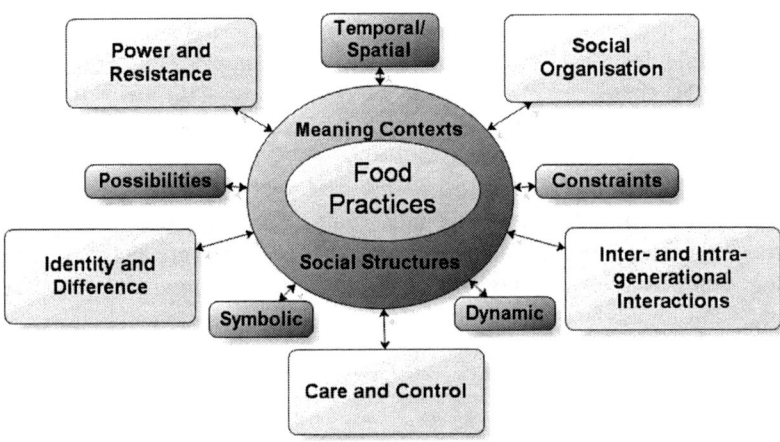

Figure 1. Research objectives.

Given the small and close knit residential community in Scotland the identity of participants and the residential children's homes was anonymised. Therefore specifics are not stated, pseudonyms are used and only a pen picture can be given of the homes involved, which have been called Wellton, Highton and Lifton. Each home provided space for six full-time residents (with one of them providing two additional spaces on a part-time basis) although numbers could be lower depending on the timing of children moving in and out. A total of 21 children (14 boys and 7 girls) resided at the three homes during the fieldwork phase and consented to Nika spending time there. At the time of data generation the homes catered for different age groups, the youngest group being 9–13 years of age, a middle group of 12–16 years, and a slightly older group ranging from 14 to 18 years. A total of 16 children (11 boys and 5 girls) and 46 members of staff (26 women and 20 men including managerial staff, care workers, three cooks, administration and domestic staff) participated in an individual interview and/or a focus group (totalling up to 12 group and 49 individual interviews plus 48 unstructured or spontaneously recorded interviews with the staff and children of these homes). The data was analysed via regular team discussions of observations and interviews during the course of data collection, a structured thematic analysis of transcripts using NVivo, the production of summaries of the content coded in NVivo, a mapping of similarities and differences across the homes, and the discussion of preliminary findings during feedback workshops with the staff and children who participated as well as the study's advisory group.

The ideal of the 'family-like' home

The family home continues to attract the attention of researchers for a number of reasons. Some (e.g. Bailey 2000) have noted its relative neglect in social theory despite the significance of the 'private', domestic arena with regard to intimate relationships, socialisation and the creation of individual identity. For others, the family home has constituted an important area of study because of the ideological assumptions associated with it and the insights that the everyday organisation of the home offers in relation to changing gender roles, ways of being 'family', and other significant societal changes (e.g. Finch and Mason 1993, Chapman and Hockey 1999, Munro and Madigan 1999, Ribbens McCarthy and Edwards 2001, Blunt and Downling 2006).

Within this body of work, tensions inherent in the construction of the 'home' have repeatedly been highlighted. Although sometimes idealised as a locus for relaxation and nurture, the home is also a space in which control is exercised, often as a way of compensating for a lack of control in other domains (Allan and Crow 1989). Homes can be designed with the public eye in mind and through their organisation they can seek to convey respectability and success (Hepworth 1999). Throughout history, the home has also been a place through which societal practices of oppression have been reproduced (Blunt and Downling 2006) and it continues to be one of the primary settings for abuse (James *et al.* 1998). As Short has noted 'the home is a place rife with ambiguities' (Short 1999, p. x) as it is a 'nodal point' of a series of polarities. For example, Munro and Madigan (1999) described the households they studied as marked by the following tensions:

> The conflict between the public, respectable face of the home and the desire to create a relaxed 'back region'; the individualistic imperatives for space and privacy and the notions of 'togetherness' and communal life; the ideal of democratic, compassionate relationships and the gender differences in responsibilities for house work and child care. All these contradictory demands create tensions that individuals seek to resolve through complex patterns of time zoning and space zoning, and a differentiation in the rights and responsibilities of various family members: between men and women, and between adults and children. (Munro and Madigan 1999, p. 117)

Despite such complexities and contradictions, the nuclear home, separated from such domains as the workplace or school, continues to be regarded as the key space for the upbringing of children.

There has long been in evidence an ambivalent attitude towards residential child care on the part of the general public and policy makers (see Kendrick 2008, Smith 2009). As Smith suggests the history of residential child care is not one of linear incremental progress but one that reflects shifting dominant belief systems 'around children and how to care for them' (2009, p. 32). Further, Smith, borrowing from Anglin (2002), describes a broad move from custodial approaches to overriding concerns with care and protection and then to more recent engagements with children's 'rights' (2009, pp. 32–33).

Current UK policy tends to favour foster over residential care and promotes the view that children need families in order to grow and develop. Institutional care can be viewed as the opposite of a family. This stems largely from an association of residential child care with images of the large orphanages and correctional facilities of the last century in which children were subjugated to regimentation, emotional neglect and abuse (Abrams 1998). Images of the 'total institution' as described in Goffman's (1961) work on asylums prevail and can leave little room for a positive understanding of institutional structures. This was certainly the experience of residential workers in the present study:

> All the anti-institutional debates that influence policy and practice, particularly in regards to residential childcare, we've had these policies and practices for years, that see residential childcare as a residual service, one of last resort, because they see the huge problematic effects of institutions (…) they view any form of institution care as a wrong. (Angus, Assistant Manager, Focus Group, Lifton)

Staff's strategies for creating a 'home'

Against this backdrop it may not be surprising that the residential workers who participated in the present study repeatedly emphasised the aim to create an environment which closely replicated what was often referred to as 'ordinary' family life:

> Because we try here to have as homely an environment as possible and with the behaviours of certain kids that is really proving to be difficult. Because you want to go away from institution and you want to almost have family life as far as possible. (Duncan, Assistant Manager, Focus Group, Highton)

Food played a key part in how residential workers tried to achieve these aims. Around half of the members of staff interviewed in each residential home made direct and spontaneous references to 'normal' life when talking about the food routines at their workplace. The generalised family home as well as the care workers' own home constituted frequent reference points (see also McIntosh *et al.* in press, 2011). For example, several care workers (such as Vinnie below) suggested things they did in their own house like the occasional weekend take-away dinner in front of the TV as a practice that could give the children experience of 'normal' family life. Through the routine of having a change from the ritual of the dining room meal to the informal TV dinner, ideas about home life could be reinforced. In this case, that the home is a space organised according to the demands of work and education on weekdays but that it turns into a leisure oriented, homely space during the weekend. The TV dinner further served as a reward for one's performance of responsibilities and duties:

> It's like the sort of thing you would do in your own house at the weekend, you'd maybe have a carryout or that. Just let them realise that this is what is normal (…) it's a treat and it's to be cherished. (Vinnie, Care Worker, Interview, Wellton)

Family life was repeatedly associated with daily and routine practices, chores and care activities such as eating together. As noted by Douglas one dominant image of 'home' is that of 'home as a pattern of regular doings' (1991, p. 287). The routines described by Lynnette temporally and spatially co-ordinate people around collective activities throughout the course of the day.

> So there is structure and routine to the day that I think resembles family time in a normal household. There's a getting up time, there's a breakfast time, there's a lunchtime, there's a dinner time, there's a going out in the evening and having your social time, there's a pick up time and there's a bedtime. (Lynnette, Assistant Manager, Interview, Lifton)

Already at the point of a child's move into a residential home food was thought of as having the potential to facilitate a sense of home and familiarity. Part of the admission process could therefore be an informal to formal focus on establishing a child's food preferences. As Rachel explained, this practice gains in importance because of the 'strange environment' that the residential home can be:

> I think if you put yourself into their shoes and you are put into a strange environment having to sleep in a strange bed, being around strange adults and strange young people and to start with it is all strange (...) if there is something that you are used to eating and you can have that it's like 'Oh right that makes me feel more at home because there's something that is familiar to me'. (Rachel, Assistant Manager, Interview, Highton)

The 'strangeness' of the building, the people within it, and the many rules and routines which governed the house created many challenges in moving the residential home beyond it being just a 'unit' for the children. 'Unit' is an official term used in Scotland to refer to residential homes for children but is also often the preferred term used by the resident children.

Staff in all three residential homes emphasised the importance of child-centred service provision and often made the point that the residential home is the home of the children not staff. The children were thought to have a right to a homely environment rather than having to live in a place marked out as different ('that's the local home' sort of thing. 'They come from the project', Rona, Cook, Interview, Wellton) or sterile on the inside like a functional public facility in 'battleship grey'. However, for the staff, giving the children a sense of ownership could also be closely linked to reminding children of their responsibilities. For example, this was the case when staff felt they were treated as 'servants', when children damaged the home or did not respect that they needed to adjust to what staff thought group living requires, namely respect, self-discipline and cleaning up after people:

> GAIL: This isn't just one person's home – this is a lot of people's home. They need to respect it for the fact. 'Oh it's only a f*** unit!' 'Well, no, actually it's not, it's your home. Where else can you go?'
> NIKA: Is that how the young people view it?
> GAIL: Some of them do, aye, and they're very verbal about that. Or, 'It's your f*** unit!' No, it's not my unit, I don't stay here. This is your home.' Yeah, I do remind them of that. (Gail, Care Worker, Highton Interview)

In addition to regular routines and paying attention to the food preferences of every child, each residential home implemented a number of practices to give the children a sense of place. Eating together and mealtime-related interactions in the communal spaces of the kitchen and dining room were considered to be key practices in this regard. They were thought to facilitate the kind of 'togetherness' associated with a family home and, again, the meanings that they carried in the care workers' own family lives could be transferred to the residential setting. In Gail's own house the kitchen was understood to be physically and symbolically the core space in which the family members shared their lives: 'the heart of the home in my book is the kitchen. My daughter's bedroom's hers, my bedroom's mine – it's not for us all to sit and communicate in – I sit in the kitchen,' (Gail, Care Worker, Interview, Highton). For others the dining room table constituted the emblematic space for family unity and care. In response to the questions 'how do you create a home?' one care worker replied 'to begin with a table, so everybody sits at it' (Cindy, Care Worker, Focus Group, Wellton).

Although across the staff group a wide variety of food and family practices were reported in relation to people's own childhoods and current lives, such long-standing European conventions around 'home' and 'family', as the ones noted above, constituted the prevailing standard in the residential setting. Attendance at the main mealtimes around the table was therefore highly encouraged in all three homes (although enforced in different ways). When mealtimes were regarded to have gone well they could accomplish such ideals as adults and children spending 'quality time' together:

> It feels more informal, it feels more relaxed. It feels like that sharing with each other round the table. It feels like they are one big, happy family. And sometimes you can actually forget these kids aren't... where they're from. It's just that relaxed. And I think the kids love it as well. (Sally, Care Worker, Interview, Highton)

Other food practices which were drawn on to define the residential home as a family-home-like space were the promotion of open access to the kitchen, the stocking of snacks in the house, giving children menu options, and encouraging children to participate in cooking and other food related chores. All justified their reasons for adopting a particular practice on the basis that it was 'child-centred'. As we move on to discuss, this child-centeredness could, however, get blurred by other objectives and constraints resulting from the three-fold nature of the homes.

The children's experiences of feeling 'at home'

The children's views on whether or not their residential care home was like a 'family home' or indeed 'their home' differed from that of the adults. The practices described by the adults above not only had the potential to create 'quality time' but were also main areas for resistance and disputes between (and amongst) staff and children. The children participated in and shaped these practices according to their own concerns and priorities.

Several children highlighted that where they resided just now was not their actual home but that their own family or community was still where they belonged: 'we've got our own home. This is not where we belong' (Natalie and Ross, both 10, Joint Interview, Wellton). Others highlighted that this did not rule out that the care home could be as good as 'home' for them but they would think of it more as a 'safe place', a 'breathing space', or a 'chill space'. Particularly in one of the three homes the children pointed out that what was good was that the staff tried to make it like a family home rather than 'what it is basically', a care home. However, what would make it more home-like for the children differed somewhat from the ideas proposed by staff. Overall, the children were less concerned with the care home being an 'institution' or a like a 'normal home'. They acknowledged that families and how they are varies. This is, for example, illustrated in a comment made by one of the boys, Ryan, when he said that eating together with everybody in his care home made him feel like they were one big family 'like the Adams family or the Simpsons' (Ryan, 15, Focus Group, Lifton), in other words not your average family.

'Institutional' aspects that the staff worried about, for example the large number of people living together or having a cook, were not, in themselves, a great concern of the children. Many said they preferred to stay in a care home than in a foster home because there are more people to interact with and the majority expressed their appreciation of having a cook. Melanie referred to the food in her previous care home as 'Pure minging, I didn't like it. 'Cause they never actually had a cook in the old place, it was just staff that cooked for you' (Melanie, 16, Focus Group, Lifton).

Across the homes the routines implemented by staff were resisted by the children to various degrees. This was not because of a disagreement over the importance of routines and the learning of skills as generally the children felt these were important. It was largely due to the ambiguous distribution of power within the residential context and the children's need to retain a sense of autonomy in an environment where they did not go to live by choice in the first place. Carrie Ann's, and others', experience of routines was that they could be inflexible and forced and unlike in your own home where 'you don't have to go to your bed at a *certain time* and you don't get to go out for a fag *at this time* otherwise your pocket money gets supervised' (Carrie Ann, 15, Focus Group, Highton).

Movement within, as well as in and out of, the home was, as in Christensen *et al.*'s study (2000), an important aspect of how the children constructed a sense of home and belonging. The first answer which the girls in one focus group gave to the question what makes them feel at home was 'going out'. The children further reported that the stringent enforcement of rules irrespective of people's circumstances did not enable them to feel at home. Melanie explained how her present 'place' made it possible for her to feel at home by allowing for exceptions:

> Here it's like sometimes it's same rules for all people, but when like some people are having a hard time you get different rules. (Melanie, 16, Focus Group, Lifton)

Other aspects that were very important to the children for feeling at home were their safety, their privacy, personal space, how their movements and access to spaces and possessions were constrained or subject to surveillance, that people help you when you are in a bad mood rather than 'leave you' or 'sanction' you, that you are allowed to have your family over.

Food by itself could not make you feel at home, 'it's just food' (Natalie, 10, Interview, Wellton). This view was expressed by several of the children. Adam made this clear by drawing the following comparison: 'there is loads'o restaurants as well, so you're not exactly gonna call that your home' (Adam, 17, Interview, Lifton). As generally reflected in the priorities of the children, what turned food into a medium through which a sense of 'togetherness' or 'home' could be created were the relationships and feelings connected to it:

> When all your family is home then you have something to eat, that makes your actual home. And at Christmas. (Callum, 10, Interview, Wellton)

> Only when my mum makes it is what makes me feel like I'm at home. (Thomas, 12, Interview, Wellton)

Many of the children acknowledged that some of the food practices had to be different because of the nature of care homes. However, there was a fine line between the staff's regulation of access to food and spaces being perceived as helpful and caring and it being perceived as constraining. For example, many children felt it was appropriate to lock the snacks cupboard which contained crisps and sweets, but when rules for handing out snacks became too rigid there was a clear perception that this was unfair: 'cause we should be able to help ourselves in our own house' (Demi, 15, Interview, Highton). The same was the case in relation to children being encouraged to help with food related chores in order to give them a sense of ownership and place. When participation was enforced, for example through a rota system or sanctions, it was not experienced in terms of learning or caring by the children but in terms of unfair control or an imbalance of power:

> Callum: 'Why do we have to do chores anyway?
> Claire: If you don't stop moaning I am going to give you more to do.'
> (Callum, 10; Claire, Care Worker, Fieldnotes, Wellton).

Having the opportunity to determine when it was right for them to participate and in what ways and retaining some control over their proximity and distance to others seemed to be important for negotiating a sense of place. On occasions when staff allowed for some flexibility in relation to where children could eat, this appeared to enable the children to feel like they were sharing power, care and control with staff; that even within the context of adult control they could have relative freedom to meet their priorities and needs, as described by Matt:

> NIKA: What makes it home for you?
> MATT: Just 'cause, there's staff here, but there's no people saying you can't do this, you can't do that. You can do what you want. Well you can't do what you want, but you can do the same things what you can do in your own house. (Matt, 15, Interview, Lifton)

Some children therefore felt they were 'coming home. To my house!' (Melanie, 16, Interview, Lifton). For the children, relationships and a sense of belonging came first, then learning and participation could follow. We will now discuss how many of the food practices associated with the creation of 'homely' environments blurred with 'institutional' practices.

The home as an institution

'Institutional' care has for a long time been associated with a set of de-individualising characteristics: the predetermined and tight scheduling of activities, the congregation of the group, the degree to which residents need to adapt to the institution, the regulation of everyday life through formal and officially assessed rules and the level of differentiation between staff and residents (Goffman 1961, Kleemeir 1961 cited in Willcocks et al. 1987). Such characteristics of the 'total institution', particularly the uniform organisation of time and space, still feature prominently in people's understandings of what it means to be 'institutional', as reflected in this explanation given by Alice, one of the cooks:

> Set rules, set times, bedtime at a certain time, up in the morning, breakfast sitting down and all sitting together at breakfast, all going to school at a certain time, wearing the same sort of clothes, your name on your clothes, things like that. It's, different children have different needs so that's why it's not good to have institutional things (. . .) like people in boarding schools, all sleeping in the same big dormitories. All in a line for their dinner, all in a line for cleaning their teeth, things like that. You don't have that in here, it's more relaxed here really. And they are trusted. (Alice, Cook, Interview, Lifton)

In the social sciences the concept of 'institution' has very broadly been defined as 'socially shared patterns of behaviour and/or thought' (Dequech 2006, p. 473) or 'particular types of conventions or practices for managing social interactions' (Mohr and White 2008, p. 488). 'Institutions' are about regulation and the normative reproduction of social structures but they can also provide guidance that is enabling (Giddens 1984, Scott 2008). The ways in which institutions are understood and put to use, Moss and Petrie have shown (2002), produce different relationships and possibilities. In residential as well as family homes there can subsequently be different ways of being an 'institution'. Spaces allow for 'action opportunities' but tend to do so unequally depending on the different positions of actors (Löw 2008, p. 38).

What overarches the institutional characteristics described by Alice above is a notion of social control from which contemporary residential homes seek to dissociate themselves. 'Nobody wants to be an institution, especially when it comes to residential care' (Will, Assistant Manager, Focus Group, Lifton). This raises the question 'how not to be an institution?' as a public provider of care for children. Is there a set of practices that can clearly be delineated as 'non-institutional'?

The top-down implementation of what were considered to be 'homely' practices by the residential staff in the present study could often be ambiguous. Equally, some 'institutional' practices, for example, the 'set rules, set times' and 'sitting down together', referred to by Alice above, could constitute justified measures for meeting the needs of the resident group. For example, the practice of providing regular meals for the children was frequently considered to be important for reasons to do with health, a sense of togetherness and caring, and meeting the children's needs for security and predictability. In an effort to ensure that these objectives were met, all three homes perceived fixed times for meals as necessary. While such a regulation of time was not specific to the externally governed home or 'institution' but was also practised by some staff in their own homes, in the residential context meals could become dominant determinants of the rhythm of each day and of what people could and could not do when and where. This is illustrated in the following interaction, in which Irwin reinforced the non-negotiability of the mealtime procedure to Marty who was still 'new' but had learned that mealtimes were the necessary precursor for being allowed to go outside:

> The meal is finished and Marty has asked Irwin if he can go outside.
> Irwin: 'What do we do after dinner?'
> Marty: 'Chores'.
> Irwin: 'So why do you ask me if you can go outside?!' (Marty, 9; Irwin, Student on Placement, Fieldnotes, Wellton)

That this ordering faculty of set mealtimes could be different from how things are done in your own house could often be overlooked, as a care worker noticed upon reflection:

> In my own house I can go the whole day without having anything to eat until teatime, so I'm not as aware of mealtimes. Whereas in here it's very much around mealtimes, everything kind of revolves around mealtimes. You don't actually notice that until you really think about it, eh? (Iris, Care Worker, Interview, Lifton)

Externally imposed Health and Safety regulations further contributed to this structuring of time as they prescribe that food needs to be served at a specific temperature. This could put pressure on everybody to come to the table quickly once food was out of the oven. As Liam explained, such practices and constraints could mitigate against the residential home being experienced as a 'homely' space in the sense that individuals or children and staff as a group could not determine their mode of eating:

> You can't really stagger these things in a unit. You've maybe got ten minutes leeway or whatnot, but the food will go cold, we'll have to start clearing the kitchen and there's so many other things. They've only got that little period – Scott's (cook) only here for so long, the food can only be left out for so long then it has to be put back in the fridge. So just from a purely practical point of view, there is only one time for a meal. But, again, I think that's... it's not really like home, it's probably more like school. (Liam, Care Worker, Interview, Highton)

Ensuring that children stay healthy and safe could also require the restriction of their access to certain foods or food related spaces in general. Duncan's explanation of Highton's procedures in relation to the kitchen space, at a time of difficult group dynamics, illustrates how a concern for safety could then easily result in practices very contrary to the original aim of creating an open 'homely' space for all:

> As a staff team we try to create an environment within which the kids have access to the fruits, have access to the fridge, have access to the kind of refreshments that they would like and would have in their ordinary home. But kids have been throwing fruits about or playing with food so we have to kind of say 'Right', then what we have to do is talk to the kids and then we maybe have to shut the kitchen between meals. You know? Food is going to be cooked away from the kids. Kids wouldn't have access to the kitchen when food is being cooked. (Duncan, Assistant Manager, Focus Group, Highton)

A similar judgement was described by a care worker at Lifton:

> The dining room was locked and it was getting quite tense (...) so in that way the kitchen can be a trigger point, it's 'I want a cheese sandwich (...) I suppose because maybe they can say Well you're denying me my basic right to eat, you know it's a different call because – had they gone in the kitchen last night they might have barricaded themselves in. There's reasons why it's 'No you're not getting in the kitchen'. And they'll tell you 'But I really need...' – my hunch was last night that they weren't really hungry, they weren't really after the cheese sandwich or whatever but if they'd gone in the kitchen they would have created havoc (...) all the knives are locked up but they can still hurl pots and pans and glasses. (Victor, Care Worker, Informal Recording, Lifton)

The examples above describe children's resistance to 'institutional' control, in this case the regulatory power of adults as exercised through rules around the use of food and 'settling time' at night. While the adults responded to such resistance with risk assessments and an adherence to health and safety regulations, the children frequently drew on another institutional standard to counteract: the children's rights agenda and within it the basic right to eat. Again marking the residential home off as a particular kind of space. In the residential context it can therefore easily be the case that 'homely' practices such as the provision of regular meals and open access to food become engulfed in a set of rules that create an 'institutional' space.

Only one of the homes felt in a position to exercise relative autonomy in relation to the regulations and laws imposed on residential homes. While the awareness of and resistance to 'procedural' practices can be a starting point for preventing constraining forms of being an institution, it should be noted that more subtle 'institutional' practices can be overlooked, for example the disempowering potential of the normative mealtime 'banter' around the table, which can function to reinforce hierarchical structures. As Higgins observed, residential institutions, in their effort to de-institutionalise their service, 'have concentrated upon improvements in the physical and organisational environment (more single rooms, more privacy, more choice, more resident involvement etc.)' (1989, p. 173). A narrow focus on such physical and organisational practices can however be problematic. Changes in relation to the organisational side of routines, by themselves, are unlikely to produce the essential qualities of a sense of home. Aspects of relationships seem to be crucial, such as being 'trusted' (Alice, above), or in Higgins words 'metaphysical qualities which go beyond the physical arrangements of place and time' (1989, p. 173).

The home as workplace

In addition to the difficulty of balancing 'homely' practices with the constraints of the 'institution' and group living context, residential homes were also faced with the atypical situation of being both a 'home' and 'workplace'. Several of the residential food practices that staff spoke about marked the residential home out as a different workplace: the issue of not getting official breaks, staff being expected to cook for and eat with the children and their colleagues, free meals, and staff's use of access to food and drink throughout the day to make up for the lack of breaks. For staff to be able to help themselves to food and eat with the children was an important means for being able to join into 'doing' home while being at work. Stop-overs in the kitchen for a cup of tea or a sandwich could be common and could aid the shifting between the different roles of managing office tasks and spending leisure time with children. As one of the care workers put it: 'That's where I think we create a homely environment from the working environment. How many other people can do that in their workplace?' (Beth, Care Worker, Interview, Lifton). Sharing such food breaks with the children and eating the same as them could further bridge between the place of home and the place of work.

The care workers in the present study explained that the shift towards abolishing separate food breaks and making meals free for staff was about the normalisation of the 'institution' in favour of 'inclusive involvement' and 'family values'. However, as noted by one of the assistant managers at Highton, there were also more practical, workforce-oriented reasons, such as getting more work time out of staff and using free food as an incentive to counteract staff turnover and recruitment problems in residential care. This highlights the ambiguity surrounding the care workers participation in food practices. Whether mealtimes count as a break or are work time was a debated issue and there were clear differences between the residential homes in regard to the staff's experience of having mealtimes together with the children. Some members of staff claimed that their own eating was not on their mind when with the children, as you attend to them and eat when you can:

I think when you're at work it's about the kids, it's not about you. And food is very functional, it provides, you know, you eat as and when, because we don't get breaks as such so there's a tendency to see to the kids first and then 'Right, OK, I'll grab a roll' or 'I'll have a bit of toast'. (Sandra, Care Worker, Interview, Wellton)

They're not [breaks], you're still working, you're still with the kids. You don't go away from the kids and your eating experience is part of the kids' eating experience. (Rachel, Assistant Manager, Interview, Highton)

In general, mealtimes without children present were considered a break from work. For these mealtimes there was often an expectation that work will not be discussed at the table, that eating is about enjoyment, a bit of personal time that needs to be delineated from work time. Mealtimes together with the children were considered work but the same expectations, namely that it should be relaxed and enjoyable for all, were still applied. There was therefore a tendency amongst the adults to use food for the reproduction of a temporal structure in terms of work, public and shared time versus not-work, private and personal time, although the boundaries between these would continuously get blurred. What could be lost sight of was the perspective of the children who were not 'at work' in the home and would therefore not see mealtimes as a break but often an invasion of their personal time.

Ambivalent feelings towards mealtimes thus prevailed amongst the staff. Several used descriptions of their negative experience of eating with the children to highlight the intensity of the work. Eating was described as a mechanistic and rushed act that could lead to indigestion. Aberrant eating was referred to when explaining the emotional and physical invasiveness of the job. Through food practices work further invaded the life domain as the eating routines in the care workers' own homes were affected by shift patterns or a perceived need to compensate for foods eaten at work.

While the adults felt that the demands of the residential home impinged upon their personal time and space, it was equally the case that workplace issues invaded what was considered the children's 'home'. Shift patterns and the administrative responsibilities of the workers largely structured the timing and definition of mealtimes and uses of food related spaces. As Matt said:

> They take up all the rooms. They do it all the time. They took in here for changeover. They took the living room for a management meeting. I said 'Look I am gonna be watching the TV'. They still took it. And I thought 'It's meant to be our home!'. (Matt, 15, Informal Recording, Lifton)

Despite the emphasis on mealtimes as 'family-like time', they were often used to welcome visitors or external workers to the residential home, in a sense, used as a 'display' (Finch 2007, McIntosh *et al.* in press, 2011) of the quality of care work delivered by the staff.

Food practices could further create work-spaces for both adults and children. They required the learning of rituals and rules of conduct. Mealtimes, in particular, could become a training ground and tester of the adults' and children's skills and discipline, either because of having to manage or cope with the exposed group setting or due to the adherence to explicit and implicit rules of conduct. From the perspective of staff the spatial arrangement of the meal with children seated around the table could also provide an opportunity to carry out focused one-to-one or group work, for example the discussion of school issues and the planning of activities:

> It's a positive thing for staff to have that sort of focus at different times of the day cause it's a good chance to sit down and discuss what we're going to do for the rest of the day or the evening or whenever we can get them together as a group. (Aaron, Care Worker, Interview, Wellton)

Mealtimes could be experienced as anxious times by the adults and children, with both becoming objects of surveillance (see McIntosh *et al.* in press, 2010). For the children this could mean that there was little distinction between the 'institutional' food practices and challenges experienced at school and the ones they were expected to participate in when they returned 'home'.

Juggling 'home', 'institution', and 'workplace': ambivalent contexts, ambiguous practices

This research used food practices as a lens to describe the difficulty of delineating social practices as either 'homely', 'institutional' or work oriented in the context of residential care. A number of factors contributed to residential workers showing a strong commitment to creating a 'home-like' environment for children and not being an 'institution'. Through their orientation to normative standards of 'doing' family, care workers were, however, simultaneously and generally unintentionally recreating 'institutional' spaces. The analysis highlights that in practice the three different spaces of 'home', 'institution', and 'workplace' intersected and could not be construed in terms of an either- or tri-chotomy. This created a context of ambivalence in which the meanings of interactions fluctuated. While care workers aimed to juggle conflicting demands and concerns in child-centred ways, their practices were often ambiguous, in that they could be read and experienced in more than one way.

This study highlights the importance of exploring children's and adults' perspectives in parallel as there were clear differences in regard to their understandings of what contributes to a sense of home in residential care. From the children's point of the view the organisational changes implemented by staff did not significantly contribute to a feeling of 'home', in fact, they may inhibit such a feeling. Measures implemented in the interest of safety or participation could too easily result in a rigid organisation of children's uses of time and space and were subsequently experienced by the children as an infringement which inhibited the establishment of mutual trust relationships (see also Punch *et al.* 2009).

Recently Vanderbeck (citing Lee 1999) argued that thinking and practice in relation to children has been hampered by 'ambiguous understandings of children's agency' (2008, p. 398). In the case of the residential home this ambiguity extends also to the agency of care workers and the residential establishment. When practical decisions have to be made, such as in relation to food, the ambiguity surrounding their agency and status can be exposed and can lead to conflict (Vanderbeck 2008). In this context of uncertainty, as the findings of this study have shown, there can be a tendency to revert to categorical thinking and the reinforcement of order in an effort to resolve ambivalence and ambiguity and maintain a sense of control. However, Vanderbeck reminds us, 'the problem is not ambivalence or uncertainty (...). Rather, the problem is that this ambiguity is masked' (2008, pp. 398–399).

The complexity of the residential home with its overlapping spheres of 'public' and 'private' and the often uneasy juxtaposition of different spatial arenas can mitigate against the creation of a family-like environment and a sense of belonging. An exploration of food practices within a residential care home is a good way to explore the blurred edges of these spaces and the experiences of children and staff who move through and inhabit them. Examples of food practices from the present research suggest that there may be no clear cut solutions. There are many diverse ways of 'doing' and being an institution or family (see Backett-Milburn *et al.* this volume, Curtis and James this volume). What seems important, however, is a reflection on the relations and possibilities that emerge from the structures that are being enacted or contested. For an institution to be a 'children's space' rather than a children's service requires the balancing of adult-defined and predetermined actions and outcomes with those initiated by children to allow for a range of possibilities (Moss and Petrie 2002).

Acknowledgements

We would like to thank all the staff and young people who participated in our research and the Economic and Social Research Council for providing the funding, ESRC award reference number: RES-000-23-1581.

References

Abrams, L., 1998. *The orphan country: children of Scotland's broken homes from 1845 to the present day*. Edinburgh: John Donald Publishers Ltd.

Alderson, P. and Morrow, V., 2004. *Ethics, social research and consulting with children and young people*. Ilford: Barnardo's.

Allan, G. and Crow, G., 1989. Introduction. *In*: G. Allan and G. Crow, eds. *Home and family: creating the domestic sphere*. London: Macmillan.

Anglin, J., 2002. *Pain, normality, and the struggle for congruence: reinterpreting residential child care for children and youth*. New York: The Haworth Press Inc.

Bailey, J., 2000. Some meanings of 'the private' in sociological thought. *Sociology*, 34 (3), 381–401.

Blunt, A. and Downling, R., 2006. *Home: key ideas in geography*. London: Routledge.

Christensen, P., James, A., and Jenks, C., 2000. Home and movement: children constructing 'family time'. *In*: S. Holloway and G. Valentine, eds. *Children's geographies: playing, living, learning*. London: Routledge.

Dequech, D., 2006. Institution and norms in institutional economics and sociology. *Journal of Economic Issues*, XL (2), 473–481.

Douglas, M., 1991. The idea of a home: a kind of space. *Social Research*, 58 (1), 287–307.

Emond, R., 2005. Ethnographic research methods with children and young people. *In*: S. Greene and D. Hogan, eds. *Researching children's experiences: approaches and methods*. London: Sage.

Finch, J., 2007. Displaying families. *Sociology*, 41 (1), 65–80.

Finch, J. and Mason, J., 1993. *Negotiating family responsibilities*. London: Routledge.

Giddens, A., 1984. *The constitution of society: outline of the theory of structuration*. Cambridge: Polity Press.

Goffman, E., 1961. *Asylums: essays on the social situation of mental patients and other inmates*. London: Penguin.

Hepworth, M., 1999. Privacy, security, and respectability: the ideal Victorian home. *In*: T. Chapman and J. Hockey, eds. *Ideal homes? Social change and domestic life*. London: Routledge.

Higgins, J., 1989. Homes and institutions. *In*: G. Allan and G. Crow, eds. *Home and family: creating the domestic sphere*. London: Macmillan.

James, A., Jenks, C., and Prout, A., 1998. *Theorizing childhood*. Cambridge: Polity Press.

Kendrick, A., ed., 2008. *Residential child care: prospects and challenges*. London: Jessica Kingsley.

Lee, N., 1999. The challenge of childhood: distributions of childhood's ambiguity in adult institutions. *Childhood*, 6 (4), 455–474.

Löw, M., 2008. The constitution of space: the structuration of spaces through the simultaneity of effect and perception. *European Journal of Social Theory*, 11 (1), 25–49.

McIntosh, I., Punch, S., Dorrer, N., and Emond, R., in press, 2010. 'You don't have to be watched to make your toast': surveillance and food practices within residential care. *Surveillance and Society*.

McIntosh, I., Dorrer, N., Punch, S., and Emond, R., in press, 2011. 'I know we can't be a family, but as close as you can get': Displaying families within an institutional context. *In*: E. Dermott and J. Seymour, eds. *Displaying family: new theoretical directions in family and intimate life*. Basingstoke: Palgrave Macmillan.

Mohr, J. and White, H., 2008. How to model an institution. *Theory and Society*, 37 (5), 485–512.

Moss, P. and Petrie, P., 2002. *From children's services to children's spaces: public policy, children, and childhood*. London: Routledge.

Munro, M. and Madigan, R., 1999. Negotiating space in the family home. *In*: I. Cieraad, ed. *At home: an anthropology of domestic space*. Syracuse: Syracuse University Press.

Punch, S., 2002. Research with children: the same or different from research with adults? *Childhood*, 9 (3), 321–341.

Punch, S., McIntosh, I., Emond, R., and Dorrer, N., 2009. Food and relationships: children's experiences in residential care. *In*: A. James, A.T. Kjørholt and V. Tingstad, eds. *Children, food and identity in everyday life*. Basingstoke: Palgrave Macmillan.

Ribbens McCarthy, J. and Edwards, R., 2001. Illuminating meanings of 'the private' in sociological thought: a response to Joe Bailey. *Sociology*, 35 (3), 765–777.

Scott, R., 2008. Approaching adulthood: the maturing of institutional theory. *Theory and Society*, 37 (5), 427–442.

Seymour, J., 2005. Entertaining guests or entertaining the guests: children's emotional labour in hotels, pubs, and boarding houses. *In*: J. Goddard, S. McNamee, A. James and A. James, eds. *The politics of childhood: international perspectives, contemporary developments*. Basingstoke: Palgrave Macmillan.

Seymour, J., 2007. Treating the hotel like a home: the contribution of studying the single location home/workplace. *Sociology*, 41 (6), 1097–1114.

Short, J., 1999. Foreword. *In*: I. Cieraad, ed. *At home: an anthropology of domestic space*. Syracuse: Syracuse University Press.

Silva, E. and Smart, C., 1999. The 'new' practices and politics of family life. *In*: E. Silva and C. Smart, eds. *The new family?* London: Sage.

Smith, M., 2009. *Rethinking residential child care: positive perspectives*. Bristol: Policy Press.

Vanderbeck, R., 2008. Reaching critical mass? Theory, politics, and the culture of debate in children's geographies. *Area*, 40 (3), 393–400.

West, C. and Zimmerman, D., 1987. Doing gender. *Gender & Society*, 1 (2), 125–151.

Willcocks, D., Peace, S., and Kellaher, L., 1987. *Private lives in public places: a research-based critique of residential life in local authority old people's homes*. London: Tavistock Publications.

Discussant piece: linking, bridging and bonding: the importance of a psycho-social perspective for Children in Public Care

Jonathan Stanley
National Centre for Excellence in Residential Child Care, National Children's Bureau, London, UK

New opportunities are opening for the child care professions especially those concerning Children in Public Care. With reviews of policy directions are calls to remember, reclaim, review and renew the distinctive child care theory and practice that was underway in the 1960s and 1970s. In the intervening period there has been something like amnesia from which the sector is only now starting to emerge. There is a rediscovery of an identity that is distinct – not Social Work or Education. For example the title of Smith's (2009) recently published book 'Rethinking Residential Child Care' can be taken in two ways – thinking anew, and also being about *how* to think about connecting theory and practice – 're: thinking Residential Child Care'.

The work by Dorrer *et al.* and Kohli *et al.* has enabled me to recover two concepts which have geographical and psycho-social connotations: 'Boundary' and 'Space'. In child care terms they were addressed extensively by Winnicott (1956) in his observations of what he called 'ordinary devoted parenting', the creation of and meaning of relationships. He was exploring what we might consider in this context to be the psychological geography of relationships, interior and exterior, psychological and social emotional geographies that connect self to others.

Dorrer *et al.* quote Moss and Petrie (2002) 'a children's space requires a balance of adult-defined and predetermined actions and outcomes with those initiated by children to allow for a range of possibilities'. This throws up a question as to the nature of current UK provision for children in Public Care: Child-oriented? Child-focused? Child-centred?

The naming of things gives them identity; the power to name defines the boundary and space. In the 1980s and 1990s for example Residential Child Care was not able to maintain its own boundary, its identity was compromised by a series of poor practice scandals. Its task became defined by those outside of it. Its purpose became fragmented as a 'scatter of interested parties' (a term used by Winnicott 1965) determined the Time, Task and Territory (yet another geographical term enters). The continuity of relationships between child and care were impinged as the lifespace became regulated by standards and inspection to which individuals and services had to demonstrate compliance.

The preceding two pieces of work help us understand that the world of relationships is always in the process of construction. It is a dynamic world, a contested space. Rather than compliance as a sign of health, Winnicott (1971) observed that it was creativity that needed to be maximised. These studies help us affirm the identity, to have confidence in appreciating that child care for children living away from home and in Public Care is a distinct field of practice. It is an activity that requires someone with the responsibility for caring/parenting to *act on* and *act with* the client, the young person. It has an essential subjectivity as Kohli *et al.* observes an act of 'linking, bridging and bonding' – key concepts for food and care.

This contrasts markedly with the world of regulation where child care activity is frequently viewed solely objectively. Dorrer *et al.* note the 'continuous construction of social realities'. What is interesting to consider is that as standards and regulations developed the consequences of objectifying relational work were arguably not fully considered. It is only now with research now that we can see the consequences of this. We achieved a diminution of role; we heightened safeguarding, but reduced the possibility of needs-led work with young people.

To be clear, the morality of regulation is well-intentioned, young people should not suffer regimentation, neglect, exploitation or abuse (and there is an ably longer list in the section 'Institutions' by Dorrer *et al.*) in settings where they come for recovery from previous trauma, neglect or abuse. However there are unintended consequences that arise and a balance to be considered. In objectifying the activity of care we made young people and carers passive recipients of others' definitions of their caring relationships.

These studies write of young people being 'active agents'. The world of regulation has sought the views of young people via *consultation*. An aspect of the recovery of the ability to think is that we are now actively addressing the *participation* of young people in their own care and welfare, including their definitions of positive outcomes. We are moving to dynamic, fluid knowledge requiring a different conception of young people's place in their own care and welfare, requiring a different methodology because of changing perspectives in the power relationship involved in Public Care.

In this re-thinking of child care we are finding unexpected perspectives useful. Food provides an insight into the complexities involved with children in Public Care. Whereas the world of regulation might have a focus on nutrition and food safety, the authors here emphasise the multiple meanings as we observe the material, social and symbolic in everyday routines. The meaning of these routines is made conscious. A focus on food is an essential for life however it also allows us to look at other essentials. A Kleinian psychotherapy perspective can augment the work here with discussions of the meaning of the breast (the first food experience) food, feeding, skin, the development of love/hate, greed/gratitude, the development of the self and relating to others.

Looked After Children, Child in Care, Children in Public Care – these are all given categories. The guidance given to workers in such child care is constrained by the formulations of the thinking behind the titles.

The concept of 'public care' has potential to become a professionalised activity rather than a parenting activity. Though we have Corporate Parents we now have Residential Child Care Workers rather than Houseparents (though we might want to critique the way this role and its practice was conceptualised in the 1970s), and foster *carers* rather than foster parents (a move that was made following theorising). In professionalising we have changed the task. It has often become a devolved responsibility undertaken on behalf of society rather than a personal engagement.

What is the idea of the use of the word 'care'? What is legitimated in the care of this group of young people? If we take a safeguarding stance and see risks as jeopardy, then how do we evaluate the necessary risk for growth, for learning, that needs to be facilitated? How does the way 'care' is defined for this small group impact upon the meaning of 'care' for the rest of the population of young people? In creating pathology in one group are we idealising the perceived normality of the rest of the population? And is this assumed normality an imported normalisation placed upon a contested space? Is there an operating assumption that there is an agreed view of what constitutes 'childhood' (a term largely untheorised in relation to Children in Public Care) and to which all children have access? Is there an assumption that by routine functioning a society achieves social inclusion – that it can be an act of delivery rather than, as the authors suggest, an act of creativity? If it is being delivered, and effectively as regulators tell us standards are improving, then those who are not benefiting (and for Children in Public Care gaps are increasing) are excluded through a perceived lack in the individual and the services for them. This is a situation that must be remedied.

Dorrer *et al.* and Kohli *et al.* help us consider where the starting place might be for the remedy. Service level or daily life? Winnicott (1986) wrote of 'Home is where we start from'. What does 'home' mean to Children in Public Care? One aspect of 'home' is a place where we are 'parented' – an essential aspect of parenting is providing a 'home'.

Parenting requires 'attunement' to borrow a term from Stern (1985). In relation to food, a parent will know when a child needs feeding, why, what will satisfy this *particular* need at *this* time, and how they must successfully provide a satisfactory response perhaps to a need the young person has even yet to register. In doing so, the child will feel *nurtured* in an environment they know is being provided in accordance with their needs. The parent is mediating the 'outside world' (another Winnicottian term 1965) feeding the world in manageable amounts. It is not challenging or asking the young person to communicate a gap felt in provision by exhibiting what has become known as 'challenging behaviour' – itself a communication that the environment is challenging the young person. Frequently Children in Public Care pause at a gap in themselves or between themselves and those parenting them. It is a matter of connection or dislocation as Kohli *et al.* observe, which can lead to rage, fright or despair. There can be islands of calm in troubled waters, an archipelago child (Dockar-Drysdale 1993), where food can provide bridges between islands of functioning (ironically white bread is often efficacious due to being very good for repeated mastication!). Left to their own devices such children will steal food so the food should always be provided by an adult. As Kohli *et al.* note it is not the consumption of food but the provision of it in a relationship. The food is symbolic of communication. Docker-Drysdale (1993), a prominent 1960s and 1970s child care theorist and practitioner, said children should become greedy for the food from an adult – for mistrustful children this was a breakthrough.

It is the relationship within which the provision of food takes place that is the central aspect of provision rather than the food itself. This is especially prominent in Kohli *et al.* where it is noted the level of preoccupation of the parenting figure is the crucial factor. Provision must involve a child receiving something connected to and reflecting their needs. Food can be a tool of communication of strife or love. To achieve this requires that we consciously act so that in every environment it is possible to achieve a successful response to an arousal cycle, to hunger for food or love. To have good attachment *practice* we need to *theorise* and the authors in this collection show how we might do this.

Dorrer *et al.* give us a framework (see their Figure 1). It is helpful as it is visual – a dominant way of learning for many involved in child care where it is the connection of head, heart and hand that will be required. In Kohli *et al.* there is a wonderful lexicon – 'a balanced plateful of evocative goodness' which may enable young people to 'have a chance to unfurl their bundled lives'. Why shouldn't theory also have a finely attuned language? 'I felt nurtured' by this language.

There is a discussion to be had regarding mealtimes in Public Care – are they an expression of adult order or authority? Is the distinction helpful? Is it any different than in 'ordinary families', where we go from demand-feeding as an infant to deferred satisfaction of mealtimes? The closeness of food and the creation of culture is clearly made by Kohli *et al.* – whose needs are being met? Fixed mealtimes do not by themselves equal reliable provision. The parent takes the authority and responsibility to defer feeding hopefully when a child is ready. It *is* an ordering of time that interferes with the infinity of infant experience and this allows for further social and educational development.

Mealtimes within Residential Child Care require that we are preoccupied with the food, its purchase and cooking. The room where it is to be served, the table, etiquette, who sits where and why, who serves and why, how each child is served. It may even require an appreciation that a child is 'pre-group' and needs sole preoccupation when feeding though they may be an adolescent – we move with feeding as with other development from dependency to independency to interdependency. The type of feeding experience needs to be appropriate to the emotional stage. In such a way the 'ordinary' is achieved by extraordinary thinking.

Feeding is about ordering of time in one regard but also about close observation and positive regard. Kohli *et al.* quotes Scheper-Hughes 'association between physical yearning of the belly and psycho-social consequences of not having food choice'. Predictability of mealtimes is important in providing psycho-social security upon which can be based other achievements. Emotional security precedes educational engagement, achievement and attainment. The provision of food is a multi-sensory experience and makes open the space for multi-sensory development. In desiring to encourage educational achievement by Children in Public Care it is important for us to learn from Kohli *et al.* and asylum seeking children that educational achievement can be lost by the 'yearning of the belly'.

References

Dockar-Drysdale, B., 1993. *Therapy in consultation and child care*. London: Free Association Books.

Moss, P. and Petrie, P., 2002. *From children's services to children's spaces*. London: Routledge.

Smith, M., 2009. *Rethinking residential child care: positive perspectives*. Bristol: Policy Press.

Stern, D., 1985. *The interpersonal world of the infant: a view from psychoanalysis and developmental psychology*. New York: Basic Books.

Winnicott, D.W., 1956. Primary maternal preoccupation. *In: Collected papers: through paediatrics to psycho-analysis*, Tavistock.

Winnicott, D.W., 1964. *The child, the family and the outside world*. London: Penguin.

Winnicott, D.W., 1965. *The Theory of the parent-infant relationship in the maturational processes and the facilitating environment*. London: Hogarth Press.

Winnicott, D.W., 1971. *Playing and reality*. London: Routledge.

Winnicott, D.W., 1986. *Home is where we start from: essays by a psychoanalyst*. London: Harmondsworth Penguin.

School lunches: children's services or children's spaces?

Paul Daniel and Ulla Gustafsson

School of Business and Social Sciences, Roehampton University, London, UK

In recent years the UK government has taken a number of steps to promote 'healthy eating' within schools. This policy initiative has, in line with the now well established and pervasive theme of children's participation, drawn upon input from school pupils themselves. Yet despite this, we argue that there is evidence of a mismatch between the agenda of children and that of adults when it comes to school lunchtime. Using data from an evaluation of changes to school meals in three primary schools in a London local authority, we argue that current policy is in danger of underestimating the social significance of lunchtimes as 'children's spaces' within the adult controlled school day.

Introduction

It has been suggested that the school lunchtime is 'a territory of contested desires and intentions; a battleground between the perceived needs of the adult and the child' (Burke and Grosvenor 2003, p. 31). In recent years school lunches have been at the forefront of the UK government's 'Healthy Eating' initiative. Yet, despite the fact that policy in this area has involved the participation of children in its development, there is evidence, we suggest, of a mismatch between the agenda of government and that of children when it comes to school lunchtime. Based upon data gathered as part of an evaluation of changes to school meals in a London local authority we argue that, for children, the government's concern with the nutritional aspects of school meals is very much a secondary issue. Unlike other work in this volume (e.g. Kohli *et al.*) which emphasise the central role which food plays in children's lives, when it comes to school meals we suggest that it is the social rather than the nutritional aspects of school lunch which are at the top of children's agenda.

In seeking to explain and understand this gap between the government's (and schools') priorities and those of children, we have drawn upon Moss and Petrie's (2002) illuminating critique of the way children are constructed in UK social policy (cf. McNeish and Gill 2006). In this they make a distinction between 'children's services' and 'children's spaces'. The former, which best describe UK policy provision for children, they see as instruments or technologies for producing outputs which are essentially adult driven – in the case of education this would be productive future workers and responsible citizens. The customers are first and foremost adults, however much it would appear as if education is directed at children. The aims of children's services are primarily future oriented:

> They are not provided as places for children to live their childhoods and to develop their culture. (Moss and Petrie 2002, p. 63)

The resultant provision is atomised and controlling; the delivery is instrumental and 'joyless'. By contrast they pose an alternative discourse of children's spaces which they see as:

> physical environments certainly, but also social, cultural and discursive... They foreground the present, rather than the future; they are part of life, not just preparation for it. They are spaces for children's own agendas, where children are understood as fellow citizens with rights... agents of their own lives but also interdependent with others. (Moss and Petrie 2002, p. 107)

Using this framework, we argue that the 'Healthy Eating' policy falls squarely within the 'children's services' ethos as we will discuss in the next section. Before we go on to do this, however, we explore some recent examples of work within sociology and geography which use a socio-spatial framework to examine children's experience of school and, in particular, the significance which lunchtime plays within the school day.

Arguably, of all provision for children in the UK, schools are the most at odds with the 'children's space' ethos. Elsewhere in this volume, reviewing recent geographical literature on children's experience of schooling, Pike refers to a growing acknowledgement that 'schools as institutions represent spaces in which children and young people's bodies are regulated through a series of socio spatial strategies and practices' (Pike, this volume). For all the rhetoric about pupil voice/participation embodied in official documents such as *Working Together: Giving Children and Young People a Say* (DfES 2004), it is clear that children see schools as driven by an adult agenda and struggle to find limited opportunities for their own agency. As Christensen and James put it: 'the spatial-temporal ordering of the school, and the teachers' paramount control over its social organisation, shape children's everyday experiences' (Christensen and James 2001, p. 79).

This is a theme we will return to later in the discussion section. If it is the case that children are highly regulated, both temporally and spatially, within the school day, what of the lunchtime? Recent work by both Valentine (2000) and Pike (2008) suggest that the lunch period is a time/space which is perhaps more contested and one which offers pupils the opportunity to create a 'children's space' in the otherwise adult controlled day. As Valentine suggests:

> Two worlds make up schools. First there is the world of the institution. This is the adult controlled formal school world of official structures: of time-tables, and lessons organised on a principle of spatial segregation by age. Then there is the informal world of the children themselves: of social networks and peer group cultures. The lunch break represents one time/space where the institutional organisation, which is evident in the way that food is organised and distributed and pupils are controlled on the school site out of lessons, is most strongly contrasted with the informal world of children's peer group cultures and the ways they organise themselves around eating and relaxing. (Valentine 2000, p. 259)

Having said this, both Valentine and Pike then go on in their respective studies to discuss the strategies employed by school staff to retain control. In the case of Pike's study the technique is fairly overt and involves 'spatial practices deployed as governmental techniques' (2008 p. 417). In Valentine's study the approach is more subtle, relying on:

> the use of food practices... to reproduce the attractions of the local neighbourhood... paradoxically therefore the school tries to control its pupils' lunch break movements and behaviour by emphasising its freedoms and allowing them to articulate their individuality through their food and activity choices. (Valentine 2000, p. 260)

This would appear to suggest that lunch is a much more nuanced and negotiated time/space compared to the rest of the school day. By focusing on the lunchtime we can see the way that different policy aims impact upon the space available for children. While the rhetoric of children's participation suggests a democratic approach to space, the implementation of healthy eating policies requiring schools to monitor the food intake of large numbers of children in a limited space and time falls more readily into the assertion of control noted in Pike's (2008) study. Whether it means that lunchtime could ever become a genuine 'children's space' and, if so, what this would look like, is another matter.

Policies on school meals

The characteristics of policies on school meals tend to be ones associated with Moss and Petrie's (2002) concept of 'children's services'. There is a commitment to safeguarding the future health of the population and aims of tackling health inequalities but despite reference to the involvement of pupils, a vision of children in the present is absent. Three trends are in evidence; a focus on nutrition, collaboration between government departments and related agencies and an expansion of spaces included in the quest to ensure healthy eating.

The incoming Labour Government dealt with the concern over de-regulation of school meals during the 1980s by issuing guidelines for school meals as they got into power in 1997 and they have continued developing policies and regulation with regard to school food ever since. Guidelines and easily understandable food groups have gradually been replaced with nutrient based standards (implemented in primary schools 2008 and in secondary schools 2009).

The National Healthy Schools Programme introduced in 1999 was a collaboration between the then Department for Education and Employment (DfEE) and the Department of Health (DoH). It represented a cross-sectoral development with a broad emphasis on promoting health and tackling inequalities. The programme paid attention to diets and physical activity and was aimed at supporting physical, social and emotional well-being in children as well as reducing health inequalities. It was followed by more focused interventions such as the National Fruit and Vegetable Scheme in 2000 where children aged between four and six were provided with a free piece of fruit and/or vegetable every day. In 2001 we saw the reintroduction of nutritional standards to school meals. The Food in Schools Programme, launched the same year, included a range of activities aimed at supporting healthy eating in schools and is illustrative of departmental collaboration and an expanding remit. Despite the broad focus in such policies, it is nutrition that is the overall pre-occupation during the school lunchtime with social and emotional well-being being less articulated.

The Food Standards Agency (FSA) has been an important contributor of advice and information to the public and in 2004 published food and nutrition competencies for children and established minimum targets for the age group 14–16 (FSA and DfES[1] 2004). They also produced the Healthy Living Blueprint for schools in collaboration with Department for the Environment, Food and Rural Affairs (DEFRA), The Department for Education and Science (DfES) and the Department of Health (DoH). This was aimed at supporting schools, reviewing standards of school meals and working with industry to improve the training for catering staff.

The move from nutritional guidelines to nutrient based standards was suggested in *Choosing a Better Diet* (DoH 2005). This was the delivery plan on food developed from the public health White Paper *Choosing Health: Making healthy choices easier* (DoH 2004). *Choosing Health* was aimed at supporting individuals in making 'healthy choices' but signalled that the same freedom could not be offered to children. Indeed children were identified as a special group requiring adult guidance in making healthy choices:

> While people want to make their own health decisions, they do expect the Government to help by creating the right environment. Therefore supporting informed choice for all is the first principle on which this White Paper is built. But we need to exercise a special responsibility for children who are too young to make informed choices themselves. (DoH 2004, p. 16)

The document '*Shaping the eating habits of the next generation*' on eating in secondary schools addresses this 'special responsibility' in its emphasis on the importance of providing children with skills and understanding, in other words, developing their competencies to choose a healthy diet (FSA 2007).

Policies have then been aimed both at the population and at the institutions charged with implementation. The Food in Schools programme (2005) is directed at schools and again sees the joint working of the DfES and DoH with an aim to support schools with their 'whole-school approach' to healthy eating. Despite changes introduced children continued to have poor diets and concerns about raised levels of obesity increased. It was recognised that a focus on the school dinner hall alone was insufficient. The School Meals Review Panel (2005), drawn from a wide range of representatives including Caroline Walker Trust, Child Poverty Action Group, trade unions, caterers and head teacher organisations, was set up to address this state of affairs by including issues beyond the school canteen. This broader sphere of interest included vending machines, the curriculum relating to food and eating, packed lunches brought from home and food available off site during lunchtimes. Public health needs, including the need to tackle inequalities and the need to measure change, were guiding principles. In order to carry out the recommendations from the School Meals Review Panel the School Food Trust was established to provide independent advice to schools and parents on how to improve nutrition at school (for further details on school meals policies see Pike, this volume).

Such an expansion then includes a number of places where children go during the lunchtime with the aim clearly focused on improving nutrition. While this is a perfectly laudable aim it is notable that an expanding sense of place has not resulted in more attention being paid to children's social experience of eating at school. The focus remains firmly centred upon what children put into their mouths as opposed to the social context of food and eating. Pike (2008) found that the nutritional discourse takes precedence over the social dining discourse in primary schools. This is despite widening the spheres included in the whole school approach as well as the involvement of the government's Children and Young People Unit. Here we see attempts to enhance 'competencies' among children whilst also supporting the school management and improvements in training for catering staff. Attention goes beyond the school gates and work with local providers in order to improve the healthy choices for pupils who take lunch off the school premises. The term 'competencies' reflects a focus on the acquisition of technical knowledge rather than a recognition of 'children's spaces' (Moss and Petrie 2002).

It is interesting to note that the manner of eating in school gets such little interest when considerable attention is levelled at family mealtimes and the importance of eating together (see Dorrer *et al.*, this volume). Indeed Hazel Blears saw families eating together as a starting point for developing Tony Blair's 'culture of respect' (Winterman 2005). The report goes on to cite parenting experts stressing the benefits of eating as a family 'are far reaching'. This is further reinforced in a report of a study of Welsh school children where the importance of families eating together is stressed:

> Evidence has shown that when children sit down around the table with their parents they are learning a lot of skills. They are not just having conversations and eating food, they are also learning about turn-taking and how to use cutlery, which helps their writing skills, concentration and attention. They are learning about morality, about the consequences of their behaviour, about society, the use of language and how to ask for more. (Brindley 2008)

However, the School Food Trust are currently looking at the experience of school meals and include areas such as the dining space, lunchtime management, promoting healthy eating and good relations. The topics identified acknowledge the constraints that many schools are working under, such as multiple uses of the dining hall, limited resources and the logistical problem of ensuring all children are fed during the lunchtime while addressing issues regarding noise and behaviour as well as encouraging healthy eating. These are issues that arise also in residential care settings (see Dorrer *et al.*, this volume) and reflect the tensions emerging in the practical delivery of a range of policies for children.

Despite the School Food Trust exploration of improving the lunchtime experience the areas identified retain an adult perspective and is focused upon managing children's activities. It takes into account many of the issues raised by children such as noise, inadequate time to eat and bad behaviour. Nevertheless the approach taken appears to emphasise a logistical perspective searching for a solution that will then be applied to this period of the school day. There is little sense that children are party to setting the agenda for the lunchtime in a way that provides them with a space to be who they are.

A similar criticism can be levied against the schools secretary Ed Balls in his pronouncement that pupils should be viewed as paying customers and therefore should be served lunch on china plates (Lipsett 2008). Although the move towards raising the standards of food and the surroundings in which these are served is a positive and welcome development, the shape of these developments are based on what adults think children should like. Children may very well like the introduction of china plates but unless children's perspectives of what lunchtime is about for them are taken into account, its introduction represents simply a further feature of 'children's services'.

The School Food Trust initiative is then reflective of many of the developments noted where children are invited to engage and participate, for example in developing competencies and through being involved with a range of healthy schools activities. However, these developments reflect a view of the child as directed by adults who have the task of ensuring children's needs are met and their future health safeguarded. Despite reference to 'whole school approaches' and 'healthy schools', based upon the intention of promoting a broad concept of health for all children, children remain atomised (Moss and Petrie 2002). The developments introduced remain, as Moss and Petrie argue: 'instruments or technologies for producing child outputs or outcomes. The child is poor, weak and needy' (2002, p. 62).

Methods

During the spring of 2006 an evaluation of changes to school meals was conducted in three primary schools in an outer London Local Authority (LA). The evaluation sought to assess the popularity of the changes introduced among the children and their parents for the purpose of informing policy development. Thus the primary motive in carrying out the study was not to conduct an academic enquiry into children's experiences but to provide information for evidence based policy development. However, some of the findings resonated with a number of issues raised in the literature on contemporary childhoods and it is these findings we discuss here. The study design relied on both quantitative and qualitative data. The former drew on available data on the uptake of school meals before and after changes to school meals were introduced while the latter was gathered through non-participant observations of the lunchtime process, interviews with children during their lunch break and focus groups with parents during the afternoon, one in each school. The latter will not be referred to as we wish to highlight the children's views on their experience.

The three primary schools selected,[2] out of the total of 43, were representative of the pupil population in the area in terms of the proportion of children receiving free school meals (13%) and their ethnic composition (50% BME). The data collection took place during a one day visit to each school during a three-week period in May 2006. The study design was approved by the multi-agency working group that commissioned the evaluation and also by our University Ethics Committee. Consent for the observations was sought from the school while for the interviews with children it was sought in two stages. Firstly from parents, by providing them the opportunity to 'opt out' if they did not wish their child to take part, and secondly from the children by asking them if they were prepared to talk to us about the lunchtime at school. They were free to break off the interview at any time.

The observations focused on the general way in which each school organised their food delivery and included factors such as the length of time taken to queue for food, the way in which the school managed pupils with packed lunches and the time allotted for each child to choose their lunch. A semi-structured interview schedule was used to guide the interviews with the children and focused on how satisfied they were with school meals, their wider relationship to food at home and elsewhere, what they thought about the changes to the menu and their views on the eating environment and the social experience of dining. Children were interviewed informally, by three researchers, as they ate their meals with their peers in the dining hall or when outside in the playground. Due to constraints of time no pre-selection of a sample was possible although the interviewers attempted to approach a variety of children in terms of age, gender and ethnicity. The interviews lasted between 10 and 15 minutes, with notes taken during the interview and more detailed writing up taking place directly afterwards. In total 68 children took part in interviews, with 32 eating school meals (we were not able to collect information on whether any of those children received free school meals) and 36 bringing their own packed lunch. There were 31 boys and 37 girls of all age groups who took part in the interviews and the ethnicity of the respondents conformed to the distribution in the schools concerned. The data analysis was conducted jointly by the team of researchers to ensure reliability.

Findings

The children viewed lunchtime positively as a space where they were able to relax, be with friends and have a break from the normal routine of the school day. Nevertheless our observations and the interviews indicated there were a number of restrictions and constraints that often resulted in frustration as the lunchtime did not fulfil its promise. Indeed it appeared as a space designed and controlled by adults where the idea of children's spaces was relegated below institutional criteria. 'Getting served', 'eating' and 'going out to play' were all processes of tension between institutional constraints and children's agency.

Getting served

Considerable logistics were behind the organisation of processing the pupils through the dining hall and ensuring they get fed. There were different queuing systems in the three schools we observed; partly to do with the facilities available to each school. Ashbrook had a dedicated lunch hall while Birchwood and Chestnut used the space that also doubled up as assembly hall, PE space and occasional lesson space. Ashbrook divided the school population into two shifts where children had playtime either before or after eating their lunch. The queues by the serving counter were fairly long and noisy. In contrast the queue in the Birchwood dining hall was small resulting in speedy service. Here each year group had a place in a staggered rota where children queued up outside the dining hall before being let in; children who had playtime before lunch also had to queue up in the playground, before being let in to queue outside the dining hall. Chestnut also staggered the children let in for lunch with a similar array of queuing systems. This began in the class room for children in the first few shifts, continued in the corridor and finally required children having to sit down at tables in the dining hall and then be called up, table by table, to the serving counter where they were served promptly.

Whichever system was adopted, children spent a longer time queuing than eating in all three schools. Clearly calm and order was something desired by children as well as adults although managing noise levels requires an important balance between allowing socialising and curtailing excessive clatter: 'I'm one of them that really hates noise because it gives me headaches' (Tariq, 6, Ashbrook).[3]

However, our findings indicated that the greater the constraint on children's spaces the higher the discontent. More conflicts were observed in the last two schools during queuing than in Ashbrook. Children in Ashbrook appeared more at ease with the supervisors and generally more relaxed and less disruptive than children at the other schools. There was also less evidence of genuine dissent among children in this school. Observed behaviour among children in Birchwood and Chestnut included willful defiance of the staff, relatively loud conversations across the halls and talking back to the lunchtime supervisors. Through observation it was noted that the structures imposed on getting served caused tension and conflicts between staff and children.

Eating

Negative reactions to the constraints imposed on getting served were also in evidence during the time for eating. Being able to be with one's friends was an important feature of this time of day for children but the seating arrangements did not always satisfy this wish. Again in Ashbrook children had more opportunities to do so than in the other schools. Here children eating packed lunch and those eating school dinners were able to sit together provided there were spaces left at the tables. It was possible to save a place at the table for a friend who was still in the queue at least at the very beginning and towards the end of the lunchtime. This was highly valued by the children as illustrated by the following statement:

> We are not allowed to sit together in class because we talk too much so we like it at lunchtime when we can sit together. (Tasnima, 9, Ashbrook)

However, during the busiest period this was not possible and children were directed to fill up the places at the tables as they had been served. In Birchwood and Chestnut children were told to fill up the seats at the tables by lunchtime supervisors and would be unable to sit with friends unless they had made sure they were together in the queue. In these two schools children eating school meals were separated from children with packed lunched. The neglect of children's own spaces is routinely evident in the organisation of the lunchtime:

> You sit with who you are told to sit with – you have to fill up the space. You are lucky if you end up with your friends. (Rosie, 9, Birchwood)

Such neglect is further reinforced by the speed required to fit all the children in during the time available. Children were encouraged to eat up, whilst also finish their food quickly. In all of the schools the chairs and tables were being put away whilst children were still eating.

Going out to play

The ability to be with and to play with friends was highly valued by the children. Having the freedom to do so would seem crucial to the realisation of a 'children's space'. As we already have noted being able to sit with your friends was something that required considerable effort and planning for most of the children. Similarly, being able to leave the table when you feel you have finished eating is also a matter of debate:

> You have to finish [your packed lunch] or you can't go to play. That happens every time. (Tariq, 6, Chestnut)

This boy felt his mother put too much food in his lunch box in case he felt hungry and the lunchtime supervisors refused to believe that he was full up. He found himself being urged to hurry up and eat up. Adjusting the speed of eating is a small element of resisting the imposition of adult definitions as is illustrated in the following encounter:

When me and Mark aren't together I just eat faster, like *[monster eating sound]* and then I go and meet him on the playground.
I try and eat quickly too, or hide my sandwiches but sometimes we aren't allowed to go after all that.
Interviewer: So what happens when you do sit together?
We don't want to go out and play so fast (Mark and Sam, 9, Birchwood)

These comments reflect strategies that sought to get round several possible constraints yet frequently leaving their efforts unrewarded. To tackle such issues through, for example, serving lunch on china plates is missing the point. The comments from the interviews illustrate how the children's attempts at agency are frequently curtailed reflecting the emphasis on the school lunch as a part of 'children's services' rather than being located in the concept of 'children's spaces'.

Not only do children hit obstacles to their plans for leaving the dining hall simply due to the duty of the lunchtime supervisors to ensure they eat enough, in some cases we found restrictions on children remaining in or leaving the dining hall being imposed as punishments.

Dinner ladies, when you speak in the line they tell you off. . . Like when she shouted at me to sit down. And she said I was laughing when I wasn't and I might have to stay [inside the hall as punishment]. (Laura, 11, Chestnut)

In other words, we see adult imposition of limits on children's spaces associated with negative sanctions.

Discussion

The theme which emerges most strongly within our study relate to the children's dislike of adult intrusion into what they view as their limited and therefore precious opportunity for interaction with their friends. Issues to do with space and time – the seating arrangements; the ways in which the organisation of lunchtime facilitates or limits their social interaction – dominate their responses. Although there are clearly school specific complaints, reflecting the different logistical and architectural features of the schools, the common theme is a conflict between the children's social value of their lunchtime and the more instrumental value placed on this by the organisation.

This focus on time and space is one which is found in a number of other studies of children's experience of schooling. For example in the ethnographic study of the last year of primary school (year 7) by Christensen and James, children repeatedly express their frustration at the fact that they have:

little or no control over how to spend time at school: who to sit by, what to wear, who to talk to, when to talk, who to work with and what work to do. (Christensen and James 2001, p. 75)

Unsurprisingly then, lunch and play times take on exaggerated significance for children as the only possible opportunities for at least a degree of control. In this study children's accounts are dominated by a:

concern with friendship at school, their seating places in the classroom and the suitability of partners allocated to them for collaborative work. Instead, the teachers' concern was to get the teaching done well and efficiently. Time for them was a key resource. (Christensen and James 2001, p. 77)

A similar picture in relation to children's concerns over time and space when at school emerges from the survey data, based on over 15,000 responses from children, gathered by the Guardian newspaper's 'School that I'd Like' project (Burke and Grosvenor 2003). When discussing time spent at school, the most striking feature of the responses is the perception among children that it dominates their lives at the expense of personal and family time. This awareness of, and annoyance at, the extensiveness of the time spent at school and on school-related activities such as homework, after school and breakfast clubs etc. is much greater than in an earlier version of the same survey (Blishen 1969). This may reflect what Mayall (2002) has termed the increasing 'scholarisation' of childhood which she detected in her various studies of children's lives throughout the 1990s, a feature which she regarded as highly limiting of children's agency. But it is not just the extent of time spent at school which exercised children in the Guardian survey. As in our study, children wanted their daily school schedule managed so that there was more opportunity for social time – for eating, going to the toilet and for interaction with friends.

In particular, the response from children in the Guardian survey on the subject of school lunches, as in the earlier Blishen study, is focused much more on temporal and spatial rather than nutritional aspects of the experience. As one respondent concluded in 1969:

> School meals are ghastly affairs, which always cause disturbance among pupils and staff (Angela, 15, in Blishen 1969, p. 150).

It is clear from pupils' responses that this disturbance flows principally from the organisational arrangements surrounding the delivery of lunches and the fact that these conflict with children's wishes for the time and space for sociability and a degree of freedom. As Burke and Grosvenor conclude:

> In both 1967 and today, children have readily associated the serving of school food with institutions such as hospitals and prisons which emphasise authority, control and the regulation of bodies (2003, p. 34)

For all the growing concern to make school lunches more 'consumer friendly' (Lipsett 2008) and despite the broadening focus in policies on eating at school, Pike (2008), in her study of school dining halls, demonstrated that the dominance of health discourses hinder considered attention to the social. She discovers that:

> [w]hile denying opportunities for pursuing social interaction, the use of surfaces to display pictures and posters in the dining room signals the acceptance of particular rationalities concerning nutrition (Pike 2008, p. 418).

Such findings indicate the lack of importance placed on children being afforded space for their own agenda. They are also illustrative of a particular food culture that places emphasis on nutrients and individual healthy choices over those of sharing pleasure over a meal. In a study comparing eating habits in the UK, USA, France, Italy, Germany and Switzerland, Claude Fischler (2008) identifies different cultural approaches to eating. Here he contrasts the US and UK on the one hand and countries on the European continent on the other, the former being individualistic in their approach to eating while the latter are characterised by a communal approach. The individualistic approach is characterised by a concern with nutrients, personal responsibility and the maximisation of choice. Where prominence is given to communion, cuisine and dishes are noted rather than nutrients, commensality rather than personal responsibility and sharing pleasure rather than maximising choice. We therefore need to be mindful of the broader cultural context within which spaces are shaped.

Locating our observation in Moss and Petrie's (2002) analysis we conclude that school lunchtimes are not 'children's spaces'. The organisation of eating arrangements is controlled by adults and driven by instrumental objectives (making sure they all get fed in an efficient and orderly manner). They are, however, contested since children see them as offering one of the few opportunities within the school day for a space within which to exercise their own culture/agency. Despite policies espousing participation for children the practice at lunchtime remains constrained from the children's perspective. Similarly, however broadly school meals policies are framed the preoccupation remains with nutrition. However, it is unlikely that a focus on the nutritional aspect of the food, be it that served in the canteen, brought in the lunchbox or by regulating nearby shops is sufficient; an examination of who it is that is envisaged to be eating this food needs a more careful underpinning as well as space to be. Consultation with children not associated with the implementation of policies at local level and viewing them as paying customers still misses the point of children's spaces.

Acknowledgement

We want to thank Robert Busfield and James Gordon for their considerable contribution to the study of the primary schools and the two anonymous reviewers for their helpful comments.

Notes

1. DfES is the new name of the previously mentioned DfEE.
2. We refer to these under the pseudonyms of Ashbrook, Birchwood and Chestnut.
3. Names have been changed in order to protect the identity of respondents.

References

Blishen, E., 1969. *The school that I'd like*. Harmondsworth: Penguin.

Brindley, M., 2008. Demise of family meal 'could lead to obesity' [online]. *Western Mail*, 23 May 2008. Available from: http://www.walesonline.co.uk/news/health-news/2008/05/23/demise-of-family-mealtimes-could-lead-to-obesity-91466-20962681/ [Accessed 20.6.08].

Burke, C. and Grosvenor, I., 2003. *The school I'd like: children and young people's reflections on education for the 21st century*. London: Routledge.

Christensen, P. and James, A., 2001. What are schools for? The temporal experience of children's learning in Northern England. *In*: L. Alanen and B. Mayall, eds. *Conceptualising child–adult relations*. London: Routledge/Falmer.

DfES, 2004. *Working together: giving children and young people a say*. London: The Stationary Office.

Department of Health (DoH), 2004. *Choosing health: making healthy choices easier*. London: The Stationary Office.

Department of Health (DoH), 2005. *Choosing a better diet*. London: Stationary Office Cm 6374.

Fischler, C., 2008. Commensalism vs consumerism – 'public' vs 'private' eating: views of food and eating in the us and five european countries. Keynote address to *BSA Food Study Group Food, Society and Public Health Conference*. 14–15 July. London: British Library Conference Centre.

Food in Schools Programme, 2005. Available from: http://www.foodinschools.org/

Food Standards Agency & Department for Education and Science, 2004. *Getting to grips with grub* [online]. Available from: http://www.food.gov.uk/multimedia/pdfs/grubgrips.pdf

Food Standards Agency, 2007. *Shaping the eating habits of the next generation*. London: FSA.

Lipsett, A., 2008. Pupils should be served lunch on china plates, says Balls. *The Guardian*, 4 September 2008.

Mayall, B., 2002. *Towards a sociology for childhood: thinking from children's lives*. Buckingham: Open University Press.

McNeish, D. and Gill, T., 2006. Editorial: UK policy on children: key themes and implications. *Children's Geographies*, 4 (1), 1–7.

Moss, P. and Petrie, P., 2002. *From children's services to children's spaces*. London: RoutledgeFalmer.

Pike, J., 2008. Foucault, space and primary school dining rooms. *Children's Geographies*, 6 (4), 413–422.

School Meals Review Panel, 2005. *Turning the tables: transforming school food main report*. London: DFES.

Valentine, G., 2000. Exploring children and young people's narratives of identity. *Geoforum*, 31 (2), 257–67.

Winterman, D., 2005. *Table manners*, [online]. BBC News Magazine, 18 May 2005. Available from: http://news.bbc.co.uk/1/hi/magazine/4551727.stm [Accessed 20.06.08].

'I don't have to listen to you! You're just a dinner lady!': power and resistance at lunchtimes in primary schools

Jo Pike

Institute for Learning, University of Hull, Hull, UK

Over the last decade the school setting has emerged as a crucial site for the promotion and maintenance of children and young people's health. Issues relating to the types of foods served in and around schools continue to dominate school health policy and occupy a central position in government attempts to avert impending public health crises expected to arise from the perceived 'obesity pandemic'. While acknowledging the ways in which school food has become a lens employed to focus the medical gaze towards the regulation of children's bodies, we need to be mindful of the tendency to regard these bodies as 'docile' and children as passive targets of school food policy. Rather, this piece seeks to problematise this view, seeking instead to develop an understanding of school dining rooms as spaces in which traditional power relationships between adults and children are contested and renegotiated. Data are drawn from an ethnographic study of four primary schools in Kingston upon Hull to explicate the contested nature of power relationships played out between teachers, lunchtime staff and pupils within the spatial and temporal boundaries of the dining room. In conclusion the argument is made that policy relating to school food is mediated by power relationships within schools. Rather than operating on static axes of power, these dynamic relationships constantly shift and are continuously renegotiated, redefined and contested.

Introduction

Geographic interest in educational spaces has, over recent years, generated a significant and broad ranging corpus of work exploring diverse topics from educational policy (Parsons *et al.* 2000) to journeys to school (Kearns *et al.* 2003, Pooley *et al.* 2005). Following calls to reconsider schools not simply as settings in which researchers might access children as research subjects, but as meaningful places in children's lives which shape collective identities (Valentine 2000). Some of this literature now reflects an increasing trend towards an examination of the socio–spatial interactions within schools and how this influences children's social relationships. Underpinning much of the work in this field is an acknowledgement that schools as institutions represent spaces in which children and young people's bodies are regulated through a series of socio–spatial strategies and practices which seek to (re)produce dominant identities and govern bodies according to a predetermined set of social norms (James *et al.* 1998, Holloway and Valentine 2000). Many commentators have noted the capacity of schools to constrain children's embodied activity using spatial strategies within the classroom (Fielding 2000, Kershner 2000, Catling 2005) within the informal spaces of learning such as the playground (Gagen 2001, Tranter and Malone 2004, Thompson 2005) and the school dining room (Pike 2008). Significant critical attention has been directed towards gaining a more thorough understanding of the ways in which children resist these spatialised strategies of power (Smith and Barker 2000, Thompson 2005) in an attempt to reposition children not simply as 'docile' and passive bodies in space, but as active social agents with the potential to construct meaning and to deploy their own spatialised strategies of resistance, albeit within the limitations of wider social structures.

The aim is to contribute to this literature and perhaps to extend our understanding of the ways in which social relationships are produced and reproduced in schools by seeking to recast existing conceptions of schools as 'an institutional space through which young people are both controlled and disciplined by adults' (Collins and Coleman 2008, p. 285). Thus, social relationships between children, between adults and between children and adults should be assessed within a wider set of social relations operating within and beyond school boundaries which are framed by classed and gendered discourses. Drawing on Foucauldian views of power the issue of school food is used to illustrate the different positions which lunchtime staff occupy within the broader social structure of the school in attempting to deliver the healthy school meals agenda. I suggest that the subjective experiences of lunchtime staff are infused with classed notions of femininity that destabilise existing dichotomous views that equate adults as powerful and children as powerless within the school.

Therefore the experiences of lunchtime staff are considered and the dynamics of power that exist during lunchtimes in primary schools. Data are drawn from a three year research project undertaken in four primary schools in a city in the north of England. The aim of the research was to examine the cultures of school dining and the ways in which social relationships are constructed and reconstructed by actors within the setting.

This piece is divided into four sections. The first section outlines the policy context in England and considers the implications of this policy emphasis for lunchtime staff. The second section provides details of the qualitative methods used during the research. The third section provides a brief theoretical discussion of power and discusses the position(s) of lunchtime staff in relation to pupils and teaching staff. This discussion considers the conflicting perspectives of the role of lunchtime staff before turning to an analysis of discipline, and resistance in order to highlight the fluid, dynamic and contextual nature of power relationships in schools. The final section offers some conclusions and theoretical insights into the exercise of power through school food.

The development of the school meals service in England

The School Meals Service in England emerged following the extension of compulsory elementary education and alongside concerns over the physically inadequate state of recruits to the armed forces during the Boer War (Welshman 1997, Gustafsson 2002, Passmore and Harris 2004). Under the terms of the Education (Provision of Meals) Act 1906, local education authorities were empowered, although not obliged to provide meals for children 'who are unable by reason of lack of food to take full advantage of the education provided for them' (Passmore and Harris 2004, p. 221). Previously school meals had been provided largely by charitable organisations and in contrast to contemporary provision 'school feeding' did not necessarily occur on the school site.

For the first part of the twentieth century, there was a large degree of geographical variation in school meals provision. Indeed, it was not until 1961 that attempts were made to standardise provision with the introduction of nutritional standards governing the types of foods that local education authorities should provide (Gustafsson 2002). During the Thatcher era, school meals were subject to a radical programme of reform which comprised a number of elements; first the removal of the obligation upon local authorities to provide school meals, except for those children entitled to free school meals; second the removal of nutritional standards governing school food; third the reduction of entitlement to free school meals through a series of welfare reforms and fourth the introduction of compulsory competitive tendering for catering providers (Morgan 2006). The latter of these reforms resulted in closure of many school kitchens as in house catering lost out to more cost effective methods of procurement through subcontracting to external caterers. It is generally accepted that this series of reforms did little to improve the nutritional value or the quality of school meals provision in England.

Typically school meals in the UK are eaten in the school dining room or hall which may also be used for a number of other purposes during the day including physical activity, assembly and worship and theatrical events and performances (see also Daniel and Gustafsson in this issue). Pupils are expected to sit and eat at tables having collected their meals from a service area staffed by catering staff and are supervised by lunchtime supervisors, who manage the eating space. Pupils who choose to bring a 'packed lunch' from home may be required to eat in separate part of the school dining room or, in some schools, in a designated packed lunch space.

Recent reforms to school meals include, the Education (Nutritional Standards and Requirements for School Food) (England) School Meals and Nutrition Bill 37, 2005 which was introduced by the Blair government and adopted a phased approach to the reintroduction of nutritional standards stipulating the types of foods that can and cannot be served at school (Buttriss 2005). Currently, attempts to improve the uptake of school meals in England, particularly free school meals feature as a central component of the government's undertaking to improve the health and wellbeing of children and young people (HM Treasury 2007). This policy area is motivated by concerns over the increasing prevalence of childhood obesity, a concern acknowledged by government through the setting of a public service agreement target to address the issue.

With unprecedented levels of media attention placed on the school meals service as a result of high profile campaigns such as those of Jamie Oliver (http://www.jamieoliver.com/school-dinners), the Merton Parents (http://www.mertonparents.co.uk/) and the Women of Rawmarsh (http://www.thesun.co.uk/sol/homepage/news/article63611.ece), the issue of school food has been pushed to the fore of the children's health policy agenda. In September 2005, the Department for Education and Skills established the School Food Trust to '...transform school food and food skills, promote the education and health of children and young people and improve the quality of food in schools' (School Food Trust 2005) and at the time of writing, government is currently accepting applications from three local authorities to pilot free school meals schemes under which entitlement to free school meals would be extended or universally applied (DCSF 2009). Additionally, the proposed indicators of wellbeing that will form part of a school's Ofsted inspection from September 2009, feature pupils' take up of school meals as a quantitative indicator for health (Ofsted 2008). Thus, the policy gaze is firmly directed at activities within the school dining room and the politicisation of school meals and its subsequent effect on the lunchtime experience continues (Pike 2008). It is the lunchtime supervisor that plays a pivotal role in ensuring that policy objectives regarding children's health and nutrition, particularly in terms of increasing levels of school meal uptake, are met.

Methods

The empirical findings presented here are taken from an ethnographic study undertaken in four case study primary schools in a city in the north of England. These case studies were selected to represent a variety of different geographical locations in the east of the city with contrasting levels of poverty and affluence using pupils' eligibility for free school meals as a standard indicator of deprivation. Ethnographic methods were used over the academic year from September 2006 to July 2007. Punch notes that ethnographic methods are particularly appropriate for those researching childhood(s) suggesting that 'it is necessary to spend prolonged, or repeated, periods with anyone in order to get to know them beyond a one off interview' (Punch 2002, p. 322). Ethnographic methods were augmented with participant observations, participatory work with children and semi-structured interviews with teaching staff and lunchtime staff. Participant observations were primarily undertaken in school dining rooms and kitchens although a small number took place in classrooms. During and after participant observations, detailed field notes were taken in which interactions between different people were noted along with their use of, and movement through, the space and the informal conversations that took place with the researcher were also recorded as field notes (see Fielding 2000, Thompson 2005).

Further participatory methods were used to elicit the views of 32 children aged between 5 and 11 years old, which included using draw and write exercises to explore perceptions of lunchtimes, mapping and photographing of school dining rooms and using plasticine modelling to communicate ideas about preferred foods and styles of eating. As Morrow (2001) suggests, using visual methods can be a means of maintaining the interest of younger research participants as well as a means of generating useful data. These sessions were videoed with the permission of participants, their parents and the schools and data were analysed thematically. These data are not reported here and instead form the basis of papers elsewhere (Colquhoun *et al.* 2008, Pike and Colquhoun 2009, Pike 2010).

Data used here are taken from participant observations, observational field notes and semi-structured interviews with a total of 12 members of staff that routinely used the school dining room over the course of the academic year. These interviews were digitally recorded with the consent of the participants and transcribed. This study focused on the cultures and geographies of school dining and as with any ethnographic research, does not claim to offer an objective account of school dining. Rather the account is partial, situated and reflective. Additionally, it is important to note that while significant classed discourses emerged in the accounts of participants, this was not the original focus for the study and was not one of the initial analytic categories developed. Nevertheless, the frequency with which classed discourses appeared in participants' accounts warranted their inclusion and particular consideration during the analytic process. Ethical approval for the study was granted through the University of Hull ethics committee and pseudonyms replace the names of the schools that participated to maintain confidentiality.

Power

While conducting the fieldwork for this study it immediately became apparent that power played a significant role in defining social relationships around food practices. Children's food practices in school appeared to be highly regimented with instructions issued about where they could sit, how they should sit, how they should eat, what they should eat and when they could leave, how they should leave and so on. The rules of the space are often written up and displayed on posters on the walls of school dining rooms. With reference to Sibley (1995), Smith and Barker (2000) acknowledge that an analysis of children's experiences of place necessarily involves a consideration of power relations. While children's experiences of schools and school dining rooms are not a central concern here, an examination of power relations would appear to be a prerequisite for any analysis of social–spatial interactions. Here I suggest that a Foucauldian view of power offers insight into the ways in which power is exercised and resisted through school food practices. I have argued elsewhere that Foucault's governmentality thesis has the potential to illuminate the ways in which socio–spatial practices encourage individuals to act upon and govern themselves (Pike 2008). Therefore, for the purposes of brevity, this current work will explicate some of the additional elements of Foucault's thinking around power that may further our understanding of the school based social relationships.

Foucault's view of power does not represent a consistent and coherent theory of power, rather his earlier work tended to focus upon the exercise of power within institutions such as asylums (Foucault 1965) and the clinic (Foucault 1976) and the production of 'docile bodies' through the use of surveillance and other governmental technologies (Foucault 1991). Foucault's theorisations of power proceeded along a different trajectory following the publication of Discipline and Punish, as he became interested in what Lemke suggests are seemingly disparate projects of the 'genealogy of the state' and the 'genealogy of the subject' (Lemke 2001). Nevertheless, despite the acknowledged difficulties in forming a consistent account of Foucault's considerations of power, it is possible to outline some of the key aspects of his thinking.

Foucault differentiated between three forms of power; strategic games between liberties, governance and domination (Lemke 2001). While domination refers to relations between unequal parties where the will of one is imposed on the other with no possibility of resistance, and government as a systematic form of regulating conduct through the deployment of specific technologies, in the work that follows, we are interested in the strategic games of power which are defined as interactions between free subjects, in which the field of action is limited by one party. Thus, where the field of action is limited there is always the possibility of resistance (Gallagher 2008). In this way, Foucault regarded power as something which cannot be possessed by individuals; rather it is something which individuals exercise and is made visible through this process. Importantly for present purposes, Foucault also maintained that power was not always a negative force but could be used to empower and to create subjects capable of making decisions within a specific field of action. Power can therefore be regarded as a productive force, in that it is capable of producing particular types of decision-making subjects.

By redefining power as something not always coercive and negative, Foucault enables us to take account of the circularity of power and the contextual and fluid nature of power relations in order to conceive of subjects that are at once active and capable of resistance in a myriad of creative ways. Additionally, his insistence upon the diffuse rather than centrally located nature of power opens up the potential for multiple sites of resistance. Certainly, by reconceptualising power, what Foucault offers here are new ways of understanding how power operates within a complex environment such as the school dining room. The following section provides contextual information regarding the responsibilities of lunchtime staff as a precursor to discussions around the dynamic nature of power in relation to lunchtime staff.

The relegation of responsibility for lunchtime supervision

Over the school lunch period responsibility for the supervision of children is devolved from teaching staff to ancillary staff although ultimate responsibility for maintaining discipline rests with the head teacher (Fredmann and Morris 1987). Variously referred to as midday assistants, midday supervisors, lunchtime supervisors and lunchtime assistants, the more commonly used term within schools is that of 'dinner lady', reflecting the almost exclusively female composition of the workforce. While catering staff producing and serving the meals are employed by catering companies outside of the school,[1] lunchtime staff are usually employed directly by the school. The average lunchtime supervisor can be expected to earn £1660 per year equating to £6.15 per hour, with senior supervisors earning around £2500 per year, and can expect to work hours between 11:00 and 13:00 during term time (Connexions). Pay, conditions and the expectations of the role vary between schools but in general lunchtime supervisors are expected to perform duties both in the school dining room and the playground. These duties range from serving and cutting up food, managing the dining room, clearing plates, collecting children from class, encouraging children to eat food, supervising play activities, dealing with accidents, supervising use of play equipment and managing behaviour within the dining room and the playground. While the financial rewards of the job are limited, the lunchtime staff in this study were motivated by the flexible part-time term time hours and convenient location that allowed them to balance childcare commitments with paid employment. Walters (2005) notes that this is common amongst part-time women workers at the bottom end of the organisational structure. Neither teachers nor lunchtime staff were asked directly about the classed nature of their work. However, as Walters (2005) and Maguire (2005) have shown, the role of lower level school staff and the role of teaching staff can be broadly mapped onto working class and middle class working identities respectively. Indeed, the 'dinner lady' has become so synonymous with female working class identity that the term 'dinner lady arms' has been used to invoke embodied notions of working class femininity to deride celebrities in the popular press (Daily Mail, 16th July 2009).

These classed identities can be found not only in the practices and accounts of practices but also how individuals think and feel about those practices (Reay 2005, Skeggs 2005). Qualitative data revealed significant differences in the ways that teaching staff, and lunchtime staff perceived, defined and felt about the role of the lunchtime supervisor. These different views are discussed in the following section.

Conflicting views of the role of the lunchtime supervisor

On first inspection the role of the lunchtime supervisor would appear to be relatively straightforward. However, teachers and lunchtime staff expressed different views regarding what the role should entail. Teachers' accounts were characterised by an emphasis on the learning outcomes that children could expect to receive as part of their lunchtime experiences. Lunchtimes provided opportunities for the speaking and listening skills learned in the classroom to be practised within the social context of the dining room and the school playground. They expected lunchtime staff to teach children life skills that would prepare them for adulthood, skills such as table manners and how to cut up food properly (see also Dorrer *et al* in this issue). Significantly, teachers did not regard lunchtimes as a time when children could learn about healthier eating. Rather what they had learned in the formal curriculum about healthier eating in Personal, Social, Health and Citizenship Education (PSHCE), could be put into practice in the dining room.

In contrast, lunchtime staff considered safeguarding the physical wellbeing of children as paramount to their role and this was articulated through a strong emphasis on children's happiness and safety as the main objective of their role. Consequently, they regarded their role as protective and nurturing and this influenced the ways in which specific practices, such as the cutting up of food, were viewed. Teachers felt that children should be taught how to cut up food and expressed frustration that lunchtime staff did not do this:

> A lot of the children eat with their hands, especially the little ones, and they do have difficulty cutting their food up, but the dinner ladies don't seem to show them how to do it, they tend just to do it for them, and then it's just repetitive, it keeps going from year to year, they just can't eat their food properly. (Teacher, Glanford Park)

However, many lunchtime staff explained that they sometimes found it difficult to watch children struggling to cut up food and not to intervene:

> At the breakfast club apparently, one of the ladies who I work with, she did the breakfast club for a good few weeks, and she said you're not even allowed to cut that bairn's[2] piece of toast in half for 'em and I said, 'why?' and she said, 'they have to do it themselves'. (Lunchtime Supervisor, Glanford Park)

In part this desire to step in and do it *for* children was motivated by the practical constraints of the space and having to attend to large numbers of children in confined spaces in a limited amount of time. Teaching children to use a knife and fork properly is time consuming and it is often quicker to do it for them. Nevertheless, what is noteworthy here is the tension between teachers' emphasis on skilling up children as adults of the future and the lunchtime supervisors' view of children as requiring protection. This reflects the competing discourses of childhood that permeated the accounts of different adults within the space and shaped the ways in which they approached the management of children's food practices (Mayall 1994, Valentine 1996, James *et al.* 1998). Significantly, these discourses are imbued with particular ideas of 'care' and what might constitute appropriate 'caring for' and 'caring about' children and young people.

Of primary concern to the lunchtime staff, first and foremost was ensuring that children's satiety was achieved. In many cases there was a perception that children were not being adequately fed at home and that the school meal might be the only meal that a child would receive over the course of the day. While this impression was gleaned from 'the little things you hear' it is acknowledged that school meals contribute to up to one third of a child's nutritional intake in a 24-hour period (Nelson and Paul 1983). This view was also held by teachers who expressed concerns for children who arrived at school hungry or having consumed crisps or biscuits for breakfast on the way to school. However, lunchtime staff also articulated a sense of obligation to parents to ensure that children received a good meal at lunchtime as the quote below illustrates:

> But they go home and the parents think they've had a healthy dinner, they haven't. 'Cos they haven't eaten it. 'Cos they've just walked out and their dinner's there and they go home and think they've had summat and they haven't. So, that annoys me, really. I think, you know, I've said, to the women I work with, no child should go home and the parents think it's eaten if they haven't. (Lunchtime supervisor, Anfield)

The idea that children might be missing out on food and going home hungry caused a great deal of distress for lunchtime staff. Many spoke of a sense of relief that children who they deemed to be at risk of going hungry were adequately fed at lunchtimes:

> If they've eaten all their lunch, then I know, when they go home, they've had their dinner and they've had seconds, and I think that's ok, at least I know they've had something, yeah. (Lunchtime supervisor, St James')

Mayall (1994) explores children's lived experiences within the school and the home setting with reference to children's agency as social actors, suggesting that children's ability to negotiate power relationships within these settings is broadly dependent upon adult constructions of children and childhood. That is to say, children are more effective social actors within the home setting because mothers are less likely to view children solely as a project of socialisation reflecting instead upon previous experience and allowing children to negotiate within the intergenerational contract. In the school setting teachers are necessarily concerned with the socialisation of children, which although couched in terms of children's independence is a project which can never be fully realised since children never reach maturity at school. Mayall argues that rather than the goal of children's independence, the aim of teachers can more accurately be described as 'conformity with school norms, both academic and social' (Mayall 1994, p. 122).

Thus, in describing the purpose and function of the role, teachers and lunchtime supervisors presented different accounts; the former based on a professionalised role with specific objectives related to socialisation of the child, the latter based on a protective and nurturing role which could be adapted to meet the needs of the individual child.

Mothering and children's practices of negotiation

All of the lunchtime staff interviewed were mothers, and all but one had adult children. Perhaps unsurprisingly, discussions around experiences of parenting their own children figured prominently in lunchtime supervisors' accounts of their own working practices. This was especially prevalent in discussing the ways in which lunchtime staff encouraged children to try new foods or to finish what was on their plate where staff employed tactics that they had used with their own children. Indeed one's experience as a mother was thought to bestow an innate sense of what the job required, and what was felt to be appropriate for one's own children within the domestic space was thought to be appropriate for children within the school setting 'cos you'd do it at home, wouldn't you, for your own bairns?'

The desire to mother created tensions within the professional environment of the school particularly where lunchtime staff were deemed to be forging personal relationships with children. This manifested itself most overtly in relation to issues of physical contact with children. Lunchtime staff were aware of the 'rules' governing cuddling children, but often felt uncomfortable in implementing these rules, especially when the contact was child-initiated. It was acknowledged that these rules existed to protect staff against allegations of inappropriate physical contact but the general consensus was that this rule could not be implemented if physical contact was child-initiated. Therefore, many admitted that they did cuddle children, particularly those that had hurt themselves but only if they knew they were not being observed by teaching staff. As Maguire (2005) notes, staff room culture often frowns upon 'bonding' with pupils.

As Mayall (1996) suggests, responsibility for the physical wellbeing of children is frequently assigned to staff of lower status within schools and reflects the greater value attributed to the former element of the Cartesian dualism of mind and body. In part, the low status afforded to the role may be symptomatic of its close associations with mothering in which the skills needed to perform these duties are regarded as innate female qualities requiring no specific training or qualifications to carry out effectively. However, in some cases, mothering skills were not seen as a valuable resource at all. As one head teacher put it, her lunchtime staff were 'just mums off the estate with poor academic backgrounds, escalating behaviour issues by shouting, with poor attitude to discipline'. Here a particularly classed notion of motherhood is invoked with all the accompanying moral assumptions around deficient parenting (Lawler 2005). It is the association with motherhood and the development of personal rather than professional relationships with children that is perceived to undermine the authority of lunchtime staff. As the next section highlights, the shifting of relationships onto a more personal footing opened up possibilities for increased negotiation and resistance on the part of children.

Discipline, negotiation and resistance

This section deals with the ways in which lunchtime staff attempted to limit children's field of action to encourage them to conform to specific conventions around appropriate eating practices.

Discipline

> ... but it's very difficult once you're friendly and matey to go back the other way and I think it would take a really long time for the dinner staff to get the same, er, the same sort of, the same sort of like relationship, but maybe they don't want that. Maybe they're happy as it is. I just think that that familiarity, it just ends up, you're just making a rod for yourself, really, cos when you say, 'no stop, I'm being serious now, stop', the children, er, they don't have the ability to sort of like change their attitude, I don't know, so. But maybe (.) but also, you know, the dinner ladies, they tend to get quite angry quite quickly, er, and aren't as measured, maybe, in their responses as I or other staff might be, so. (Teacher, Anfield)

In general teaching staff regarded lunchtime staff as well meaning but lacking the necessary skills to maintain discipline and order. As Lawler points out, working class women are frequently constituted and reconstituted as 'lacking' in relation to middle class motherhood and middle class women are constantly required to distance and distinguish themselves from the working class in a bid to maintain their subjective status (Lawler 2002). In the quote above it is the familiarity of the relationship between lunchtime staff and the children that is cited as the reason that discipline and order is not maintained over lunchtime. However, it was also clear that teachers regarded the ability to maintain order and discipline as something intrinsic, stemming from an innate ability to command respect and a product of their individual ontology. For example, in what follows a teacher discusses her preferred approach to managing seating and queuing arrangements in the dining room and how effective this would be in maintaining pupil discipline:

> Q: So do you think that's because you're trained as a teacher, that you know what to do with them?
> A: No, I think it's because of my views.

It is worth noting that while teachers receive a great deal of training in classroom management and other aspects of behaviour and discipline, there is no formal training for lunchtime staff who may be responsible for up to 75 children at a time in an environment which is far less structured than the classroom. Despite this lack of training and the larger number of pupils under their care, many teachers felt that lunchtime staff simply had a different view of children and this accounted for their failure to maintain order. While lunchtime staff acknowledged the difficulties in maintaining order, they were more likely to attribute this to structural and organisation factors such as the increased ratio of pupils to staff over the lunchtime period, the lack of respect for lunchtime staff and the limited sanctions that they were able to apply when pupils behaved inappropriately. Increased ratios meant that lunchtime staff could not undertake effective surveillance to ensure order was maintained, the lack of respect meant that they were challenged more often than teachers and the limited sanctions meant that they had to rely on the support of teaching staff to implement these sanctions. In the majority of cases, lunchtime staff did not feel that they received adequate support from teachers regarding the enforcement of punishments for inappropriate behaviour. These factors were summed up with the often-repeated phrase 'I don't have to listen to you, you're just a dinner lady'.

Negotiation

Holt (2004) notes that while teachers are involved in more authoritarian disciplinary practices, ancillary staff such as classroom assistants practice less overt strategies of power. However, as Gallagher (2008) suggests this may be the result of pupils' more sophisticated practices of resistance. Lunchtime staff in this study exercised a variety of techniques through which to encourage, persuade and cajole children to conform to expectations around food:

> You use bribery, well, not bribery, that's not the right word, you manipulate, don't you? I mean, like [name] today, he's been told that if he doesn't eat his lunch (...) they're given choices and they know the choices. (Lunchtime supervisor, St James')

The choices given to pupils in this context inevitably limit pupils' field of action. Thus the choice amounts to pupils' conformity with expected norms, or their acceptance of designated punishments. Nevertheless, many of the negotiations around food practices were more subtle than this and involved considerable flexibility on the part of both lunchtime staff and pupils to arrive at agreed solutions, for example, jacket potatoes were eaten as long as the skin was removed, apples would be consumed when they were cut into pieces and pupils would agree to eating one more mouthful if they could then leave the dining room afterwards.

Other methods of encouragement included the awarding of stickers or other special privileges if pupils conformed to expected conventions around food. These included awarding house points, golden tickets and spaces on the golden table. The golden table or top table had a table cloth and often flowers and special beakers and plates. Pupils that had behaved particularly well in the dining room by eating all their dinner, trying something new or exhibiting good table manners, for example, were able to sit on the special table with their invited guests. As Holt points out these methods can be regarded as disciplinary techniques 'that reward children for achieving expected norms of learning or bodily performance' (Holt 2004, p. 20)

Lunchtime staff were certainly aware that persuasion and encouragement were the only methods available to them and that once these were exhausted, it was children that possessed ultimate power and control over what they wished to eat.

> But I mean, I like send them back once, but if they say they really, really don't like it then, I think, well I'm not gonna sit and force 'em to eat it if it's something they don't like, you know? (Lunchtime supervisor, Upton Park)

Resistance

Where practices of negotiation failed, the authority of lunchtime staff was challenged in three ways: by avoiding surveillance; ignoring lunchtime staff or confronting them directly. The most frequently deployed strategy was to avoid the surveillance of the lunchtime staff in an attempt to get to the waste bin and deposit unwanted food. In some cases pupils would make two or three forays before being successful:

> He went up for seconds! Apparently, I didn't see, but apparently he was being cheeky behind my back, but I didn't know that, so. But if I'd seen that, that's when he would've got time-out, I'd have said 'no I'm not taking that'. (Lunchtime supervisor, St James')

This was supported by observational data as the following extract from field notes illustrates:

> There appears to be a route that children take when they want to sneak to the bin. It's right past me on the right hand side of the dining room in between the tables and the wall and then there is a bit of gym equipment to squeeze past to get to the bin. This route is the one which takes you furthest away from where the lunchtime supervisor stands in the dining room. Especially if she is down at the other end, away from the bin. (Field notes, Upton Park)

The peripheries of the dining room were often used to escape the surveillance of lunchtime staff as these were the least visible parts of the room. As previously stated, many dining spaces were also used in the morning and afternoon for physical activity, dramatic performances, assembly and worship. Consequently, dining spaces were frequently cluttered with crash mats, benches, climbing ropes and gym equipment, musical instruments and theatrical equipment and staging which fostered greater opportunities for avoiding surveillance and subversion. Nevertheless, this was something that lunchtime staff were aware of and tried to monitor.

The requests of lunchtime staff were frequently ignored. Field notes demonstrate children being asked to comply with the rules of the dining room with varying levels of success. This was notable in terms of seating arrangements and correct bodily deportment.

> A lunchtime supervisor tries to direct a boy to a table. He has just entered the dining room with his flight tray and he is walking towards the right hand side of the dining room. She shows him a place on the left hand side of the dining room. He ignores this and goes off to the seat he had originally intended on the right hand side. (Field notes, Glanford Park)

This strategy tended to be employed in the busier dining rooms where lunchtime staff were busy and easily distracted by other tasks. Thus, requests for compliance were rarely followed up. Finally, the least frequent strategy observed was directly challenging the authority of lunchtime staff. Lunchtime staff reported being hit, kicked, having fingers bent back, being called names, being spat at and sworn at by children. In one school, rules regarding conduct in the dining room were frequently flouted as children defined their own expectations around bodily conduct. Attempts to regulate the space often failed in the face of direct challenges from children.

> A boy on the pack up table launches a package at the bin and successfully lands it! A girl next to the pack up table is trying to climb up the pipes on the wall. A boy in the middle of the dining room is pretending to be an aeroplane. He is challenged by the lunchtime supervisor and he just shouts at her. (Field notes, Glanford Park)

In this school some children reported finding this environment chaotic and threatening with expectations around appropriate behaviour inconsistently implemented. Indeed, this view would support the Foucauldian view that power can be exercised in a positive and protective way that in this instance might have resulted in children feeling safer and more comfortable in the space.

Conclusion

The above has illustrated some of the ways in which power plays out in the increasingly politicised space of English primary school dining rooms. It has explored the divergent approaches of lunchtime staff and teaching staff in relation to pupils' practices of food and eating and has highlighted the contentious and dynamic nature of power relationships, eschewing the traditional depiction of adults within schools as a homogenous and powerful group. Rather than equating adults with positions of power and children as disciplined bodies within school spaces, I suggest that lunchtime staff are constructed as deficient against the norm of professional middle class teachers. This construction and reconstruction through practices of food and eating is inscribed with classed and gendered discourses that exist beyond the boundaries of the school and are bound up with classed notions of childrearing and motherhood. This perceived deficiency opens up spaces for children to forge different relationships with lunchtime staff that resonate with Foucault's conceptions of strategic games between liberties and the circularity of power. While in some instances this results in closer and more personal relationships between lunchtime staff and pupils, it also frequently leads to confrontations as rules are negotiated and contested with more or less force. Indeed, pupils may be well aware of the internal hierarchies that operate within schools and fully cognisant of the limits of the authority of lunchtime staff. Thus they may be entirely reasonable in the assertions that 'I don't have to listen to you, you're just a dinner lady'.

Acknowledgements

With thanks to Professor Derek Colquhoun for his support and advice and to the lunchtime staff and schools that took part in this research. Thanks also to Ian McIntosh and the two anonymous reviewers for their comments on an earlier draft.

Notes

1. While a small number of schools have taken catering in house, the majority are supplied by large catering companies or local authorities.
2. Bairns is a colloquial term for children.

References

Board of Education, 1906. *Education (provision of meals) act*. London: HMSO.
Buttriss, J., 2005. Government promises school meals will be transformed. *Nutrition Bulletin*, 30 (3), 211–214.
Catling, S., 2005. Children's personal geographies in the English primary school geography curriculum. *Children's Geographies*, 3, 325–344.
Collins, D. and Coleman, T., 2008. Social geographies of education: looking within and beyond school boundaries. *Geography Compass*, 2, 281–299.
Colquhoun, D., Wright, N., Pike, J., and Gatenby, L., 2008. *Evaluation of 'Eat well do well', Kingston-upon-Hull's school meal initiative*, [online]. Available from: http://www2.hull.ac.uk/IFL/pdf/IFL-R_finalreport.pdf [Accessed 30 November 2009].
Connexions, *School lunchtime supervisor*, [online]. Available from: http://www.connexions_direct.com/Jobs$U/index.cfm?pid=47&catalogueContentID=155 [Accessed 28 April 2009].

Daily Mail., Available from: http://wwwdailymail.co.uk/tvshowbiz/article-1199849/Is-Madonna-losing-arms-race-Singer-reveals-bingo-wings-night-Italy.html

DCSF, 2009. *Local Authorities to bid for free school meal pilots* [online]. Available from: http://www.dcfs.gov.uk/pns/DisplayPN.cgi?pn_id=2009_0010 [Accessed 28 April 2009].

Fielding, S., 2000. Walk on the left! Children's geographies and the primary school. *In*: S. Holloway and G. Valentine, eds. *Children's geographies: playing, living, and learning*. Routledge: London.

Foucault, M., 1965. *Madness and civilisation: a history of insanity in the age of reason*. New York: Random House.

Foucault, M., 1976. *The birth of the clinic: an archaeology of medical perception*. Hants: Tavistock.

Foucault, M., 1991. *Discipline and punish: the birth of the prison*. London: Penguin.

Fredmann, S. and Morris, G., 1987. The teachers' lesson: collective bargaining and the courts. *Industrial Law Journal*, 16, 215–226.

Gagen, E.A., 2001. Too good to be true: representing children's agency in the archives of the playground movement. *Historical Geography*, 29, 53–64.

Gallagher, M., 2008. Foucault, power and participation. *International Journal of Children's Rights*, 16, 395–406.

Gustafsson, U., 2002. School meals policy; the problem with governing children. *Social Policy and Administration*, 36, 685–697.

Harris, B., 1995. Educational reform, citizenship and the origins of the school medical service. *In*: M. Gijswijt-Hofstra and H. Marland, eds. *Cultures of child health in britain and the netherlands in the twentieth century*. Amsterdam: Rodopi, 85–101.

Holloway, S. and Valentine, G., 2000. Children's geographies and the new social studies of childhood. *In*: S. Holloway and G. Valentine, eds. *Children's geographies: playing, living, learning*. London: Routledge.

Holt, L., 2004. The 'Voices' of children: de-centring empowering research relations. *Children's Geographies*, 2 (1), 13–27.

HM Treasury, 2007. *PSA delivery agreement 12: improve the health and wellbeing of children and young people*. London: HMSO.

James, A., Jenks, C., and Prout, A., 1998. *Theorising childhood*. Cambridge: Polity Press.

Kearns, R., Collins, D., and Neuwelt, P., 2003. The walking school bus: extending children's geographies? *Area*, 35 (3), 285–292.

Kershner, R., 2000. Organising the physical environment of the classroom to support children's learning. *In*: D. Whitebread, ed. *The psychology of teaching and learning in the primary school*. London: Routledge Falmer.

Lawler, S., 2002. Mobs and monsters: independent man meets Paulsgrove woman. *Feminist Theory*, 3, 103–113.

Lawler, S., 2005. Disgusted subjects: the making of middle-class identities. *The Sociological Review*, 53 (3), 429–446.

Lemke, T., 2001. The birth of bio-politics': Michel Foucault's lecture at the College de France on neo-liberal governmentality. *Economy and Society*, 30 (2), 190–207.

Maguire, M., 2005. Textures of class in the context of schooling: the perceptions of a 'class-crossing' teacher. *Sociology*, 39 (3), 427–443.

Mayall, B., 1994. Children in action at home and school. *In*: B. Mayall, ed. *Children's childhoods observed and experienced*. London: Routledge Falmer.

Mayall, B., 1996. *Children, health and the social order*. Buckingham: Open University Press.

Morgan, K., 2006. School food and the public domain: the politics of the public plate. *Political Quarterly*, 77 (3), 379–387.

Morrow, V., 2001. Using qualitative methods to elicit young people's perspectives on their environments: some ideas for community health initiatives. *Health Education Research, Theory and Practice*, 16 (3), 255–268.

Nelson, M. and Paul, A.A., 1983. The nutritive contribution of school dinners and other midday meals to the diets of schoolchildren. *Human Nutrition: Applied Nutrition*, 37A, 128–135.

Ofsted, 2008. *Indicators of a school's contribution to wellbeing consultation document*. London: Ofsted.

Parsons, E., Chalkley, B., and Jones, A., 2000. School catchments and pupil movements: A case study in parental choice. *Educational Studies*, 26 (1), 33–48.

Passmore, S. and Harris, G., 2004. Education, health and school meals: a review of policy changes in England and Wales over the last century. *Nutrition Bulletin*, 29 (3), 221–227.

Pike, J., 2008. Foucault, space and primary school dining rooms. *Children's Geographies*, 6 (4), 413–422.

Pike, J., forthcoming 2010. *An ethnographic study of primary school dining rooms*, Unpublished thesis. University of Hull.

Pike, J. and Colquhoun, D., 2009. The relationship between policy and place: the role of school meals in addressing health inequalities. *Health Sociology Review*, 18 (1), 50–60.

Pooley, C.G., Turnbull, J., and Adams, M., 2005. The journey to school in Britain since the 1940s: continuity and change. *Area*, 7 (1), 43–53.

Punch, S., 2002. Research with children: the same or different from research with adults? *Childhood*, 9 (3), 321–341.

Reay, D., 2005. Beyond consciousness? The psychic landscape of social class. *Sociology*, 39 (5), 911–928.

School Food Trust, 2005, Available from: http://www.schoolfoodtrust.org.uk/index.asp

Skeggs, B., 2005. The making of class and gender through visualizing moral subject formation. *Sociology*, 39 (5), 965–982.

Smith, F. and Barker, J., 2000. Contested spaces: children's experiences of out of school care in England and Wales. *Childhood*, 7 (3), 315–333.

Thompson, S., 2005. 'Territorialising' the primary school playground: deconstructing the geography of playtime. *Children's Geographies*, 3 (1), 63–78.

Tranter, P. and Malone, K., 2004. Geographies of environmental learning: an exploration of children's use of school grounds. *Children's Geographies*, 2 (1), 131–155.

Valentine, G., 1996. Angels and devils: moral landscapes of childhood. *Environment and Planning D*, 14, 581–599.

Valentine, G., 2000. Exploring children and young people's narratives of identity. *Geoforum*, 31, 257–267.

Walters, S., 2005. Making the best of a bad job? Female part-timers' orientations and attitudes to work. *Gender, Work & Organization*, 12 (3), 193–216.

Welshman, J., 1997. School meals and milk in England and Wales. 1906–45. *Medical History*, 41, 6–29.

Discussant piece: food and schools

Ian McIntosh, Ruth Emond and Samantha Punch
Department of Applied Social Science, University of Stirling, Stirling, Scotland

The school has long been regarded as having responsibility for not only the intellectual development of children but also their social and physical wellbeing. As such the school has become one of the most externally surveyed and regulated spaces that children and adults pass through. This is particularly the case in relation to adult's and children's food and their accompanying food practices. The school has thus been central in policy interventions in children's lives through the supply of various food substances (milk, fruit, free school meals) as well as attempts to develop the expected social norms that revolve around and through food practices (e.g. sitting at the table, sharing, serving food etc.) (Dickie 2004). Indeed schools are often seen to be a key social institution through which to supplement, or indeed, counteract food experiences and practices that children may have at home; a space in which they can supervised and monitored in ongoing efforts to instil 'good' habits and be made to eat the 'right' sort of food (McKendrick 2004a, 2004b, Kime 2008). The preceding two studies emphasise this point that schools are regarded within social policy as an important site to change and influence eating behaviours, in particular, as Daniel and Gustafsson note, with a current emphasis on school as a place where children's nutritional intake is monitored (Cunningham 2003, see also Dickie 2004 on the school meals in Scotland). School mealtimes have therefore become not only a training ground for children for the learning of life-skills, morality and manners but a way to improve their health and wellbeing. Indeed, as Pike notes, 'school dinners' have become incredibly newsworthy and seem to carry a great weight of popular expectation in relation to improving the nation's health and the health of future generations. This is of course particularly the case with current Government concerns and media obsessions with 'obesity' (see Proctor *et al.* 2008). To this extent, as Pike points out, school dinners have become highly politicised.

What is of particular interest in the preceding two pieces is the way in which these large, governed institutions share many of the tensions and fraught exchanges around food with families and other smaller care based institutions (Kime 2008). In social spaces such as schools, where the needs of many must be balanced with the needs of the individual, it can be difficult to assess the impact that food and food practices can have on children, as well as many of the other powerfully symbolic uses of food that are explored in this collection. The dinner hall and school meals generally, as the authors detail, can be sites which involve interweaving asymmetries of power and where classed and gendered discourses are played in a complex ebb and flow of resistance and incorporation. In this way, food often acts as medium through which there is a coming together of formal and informal codes and social mores thus adults and children alike (re)create spaces within formalised sites such as the school where they can assert their own rituals and norms (McKendrick 2004a). As Daniel and Gustafsson suggest, as far as children are concerned, it is the social rather than the nutritional aspects of school lunch that are paramount.

Pike, in her study of school dinners across four primary schools, explores the ways in which power, in relation to its distribution, enforcement, negotiations and links to identity, was significantly played out around food. In the schools she studied a clear hierarchy was evident which placed management staff above teaching staff and similarly teaching staff above the women, 'Dinner Ladies', involved in the direct supply or monitoring of children's food and food related behaviours. Interweaving discourses of class and gender were evident as adults sometimes clashed for the 'correct' set of practices to impart to the children in their care. In addition, Pike outlines the ways in which children developed relations with dinner ladies which reflected prevailing assumptions about class, gender and authority.

What comes across clearly from both studies is the social and spatial nature of food and food practices. How food is managed and experienced can not be dislocated from the construction of 'normal' eating behaviours, skills and taste. The origin and legitimacy of such norms are complex and often not shared by both those giving and monitoring food in schools and those receiving it. The school dinner-time is thus a space and time of contestation and sees daily struggles over ownership of that particular space and time and the behaviours that take place within and during it. The fundamental question that both authors raise for discussion then is precisely who and what is the school dinner for?

Space and interactions are constituted, in part, through networks of power and for children lunch-times and dinner halls can be spaces where they can exert a greater degree of agency than is possible during the rest of the normal school day. The extent to which this is resisted and seen by adults as legitimate is discussed in both pieces of research and the consequences of this for developing an effective policy in relation to current norms of 'healthy eating' and promoting agendas of children's participation (Daniel and Gustafsson) in relation to schools and food is explored in a way that is both revealing and important.

References

Cunningham, C., 2003. A fruitful direction for research in children's geography: fat chance? *Children's Geographies*, 1 (1), 125–127.

Dickie, J, 2004. Tackling child food poverty in Scotland through universal school meals provision. *Children's Geographies*, 2 (2), 287–295.

Kime, N., 2008. Children's eating behaviours: the importance of the family setting. *Area*, 40 (3), 315–322.

McKendrick, J., 2004a. The diet of children's geographies. *Children's Geographies*, 2 (2), 287–295.

McKendrick, J., 2004b. Fallacies surrounding the geography of family eating. *Children's Geographies*, 2 (2), 293–295.

Proctor, K.L., Clarke, G.P., Ransley, J.K., and Cade, J., 2008. Micro-level analysis of childhood obesity, diet, physical activity, residential socioeconomic and social capital variables: where are the obesogenic environments in Leeds? *Area*, 40 (3), 323–340.

Children's snacking, children's food: food moralities and family life

Penny Curtis[a], Allison James[b] and Katie Ellis[c]

[a]School of Nursing and Midwifery, University of Sheffield, Sheffield, UK; [b]Department of Sociological Studies, University of Sheffield, Sheffield, UK; [c]Interdisciplinary Centre of the Social Sciences, University of Sheffield, Sheffield, UK

This work considers the construction of *children's* food and *children's* eating practices, in the narratives of children, aged 11–12, and their parents, and explores what these constructions reveal about child–adult relations and the nature of family life. It argues that, implicit to the differentiation of children's and adult's food and eating practices within families are generationally nuanced food moralities. We suggest that the day-to-day, ongoing negotiation and management of these generationally nuanced food moralities is integral to the constitution of intergenerational relations and generational identity and, indeed, the idea of 'family' itself.

Introduction

Criticisms of British children's eating practices are so widespread as to be commonplace, almost every-day, occurrences. On the one hand, children themselves are criticised for their apparent inability and unwillingness to make 'sensible' eating choices while, on the other, they are portrayed as the victims of irresponsible parenting practices. In 2006, for example, under the headline 'British children eat 825 snacks per year', the tabloid newspaper *The Mail*, proclaimed that:

> Snacking is so ingrained in UK eating habits that it has become a way of life rather than a 'trend' – a 'way of life', for British children, that marks 'society's move away from traditional sit-down meals' and the eating of proper food (The Mail 2006[1]).

Advice currently promulgated by the NHS Change 4 Life campaign[2] echoes this alarm. It advises both that snacks are often high in 'all the things we shouldn't eat too much of'[3] and that children and parents 'should eat together when they can' since this shared practice is assumed to strengthen 'the family bond'.[4]

Such public concerns are intriguing for, embedded within them, are not only moralities about specific foods – the distinctions, for example, between good and bad food, proper and (by implication) improper food – but also specific moralities about how family life should be. The latter is apparent in the quotation above: through their improper eating practices, children may be challenging or, indeed, threatening family relationships. Their consumption of snacks and their reported propensity for eating on the go, promise to undermine family life since such eating practices stand in contradistinction to the proper food consumed at a shared family meal which is held to signal the togetherness of the family (Murcott 1983, Charles and Kerr 1988, Devault 1994). However, as we have shown elsewhere, such moral panics are unjustified since these 'new' food practices of children are not necessarily having detrimental effects on 'the family' (James *et al.* 2009). Even if snacking has become ingrained in UK eating habits, the notion of proper food that is eaten together still retains its iconic status as a symbol of what a proper family does. In short, then, the challenge to traditional food and eating practices and to family life that children's snacking and grazing are held to represent may not, in fact, be taking place, despite populist claims to the contrary. In the following we explore why this might be so.

Proper food and proper family life

A proper meal has been argued to be one that contains proper food requiring time and effort to prepare: it uses ingredients that are 'fresh' and 'natural' and which are cooked and served hot (Charles and Kerr 1988, Willets 1997). Proper food is, suggest Bell and Valentine (2003), that which is considered 'good food', and in the mid to late twentieth century, proper food in the UK came together in a particular cultural form as the quintessential family meal of meat, potato and vegetables (Murcott 1983, Willets 1997). However, although more recent research has shown that what constitutes proper food is contextually specific (Blake *et al.* 2009) and indeed that the content of the family meal has become less stable over historical time, nonetheless many families – and particularly mothers, who continue to carry the majority of responsibility for provisioning and feeding in the family – retain a commitment to cooking proper food. And they do so even if the exigencies of modern life mean that their ability to realise this ideal on a day-to-day basis may be heavily constrained (James *et al.* 2009). Thus, although the meal of 'meat, potato and vegetable' may have lost its ubiquity in the UK, as family meals have accommodated a wider variety of foodstuffs and new food practices (Silva and Smart 2004, Smart 2007, Curtis *et al.* 2009), the symbolic significance of 'proper food' and the 'proper family meal' has endured.

While proper food is thus core to the proper meal and proper family life, the meaning bearing significance of the 'proper family meal' lies not just in the configuration of the foods that are made available to family members. Critically, it also encompasses the practices that are inferred and enabled such that the family meal is consumed in an act of togetherness, providing 'moments of intersection' for family members (Smart 2007, p.170). As Lupton (1996, p. 39) notes:

> It is not necessarily the food that is served at family meals that is considered important, but the ritual of sitting down to eat the meal. The 'family meal' and the 'dinner table' are potent symbols, even metonyms of the family itself.

The cultural value accorded to such rituals is interesting, given that recent work indicates that the construction of the family meal as a 'universal, regularly practised, stable event' is largely an historical myth (Jackson *et al.* 2009, p. 144). Yet this myth of the proper family coming together to eat a proper family meal is, as Murcott (1983) notes, part and parcel of the ideology of the family. If the preparation and consumption of a family meal helps to define and constitute family *as* a family (Devault 1994, Morgan 1996), then proper families (at least aspire to) eat proper food, prepared with care and consumed in an act of togetherness (Murcott 1983, Lupton 1996, James *et al.* 2009). The metonyms of the 'family meal' and the 'dinner table' remain as a powerful normative presence in family life, even when family members cannot or do not sit together around a dinner table. Indeed, the importance of the family meal remains deeply ingrained in contemporary food discourses. Whether eaten in the public domain of the restaurant (Brembeck 2005) or within the privacy of the family home, family members sitting together to eat a family meal has come to be seen as a virtuous undertaking which strengthens family life, as Green *et al.* (2009) have shown in their study of community-based food programmes in the UK. The ritual of the family meal continues, therefore, to provide family members with a 'stable, reassuring family [they] can live by' (Gillis 1996, p. 15).

Jackson (2009, p. 10) notes, however, that the making and eating of proper family meals is 'a widely shared (middle-class) aspiration', an observation that deserves further comment, since food consumption and eating practices have been shown to be strongly influenced by socio-economic factors, with socio-economically disadvantaged families eating less 'healthy' diets than those in more advantaged socio-economic circumstances (Shaw *et al.* 2000, Sproston and Primatesta 2003, Crawford and Jeffery 2005, Wills *et al.* 2008). Indeed, in this issue, Backett-Milburn *et al.* suggest that the eating practices of teenagers in middle class and working class families are closely tied to families' socio-economic circumstances, albeit in rather different ways. Thus, in determining what teenagers eat, class matters. While for working class young people, economic constraints mean that they have little control over the foods provided, Backett-Milburn *et al.* (this issue) argue that the control exerted by young people in middle class families is similarly restricted: in this case, parents work to mould eating practices and tastes in the making of future middle class adults.

However, in the discussion that we develop here, we are not so much concerned with precisely what foods family members do, or do not eat, as part of their family meal. Nor are we concerned with which foodstuffs are, or are not, considered by different kinds of families to be 'improper' snacks, as opposed to the 'proper' ingredients of a meal. Instead, we explore the ways in which such cultural conceptions and distinctions are employed and how they are negotiated between familial generations. And, in this respect at least, the empirical data to be discussed in this piece cannot be best accounted for in terms of social class. Rather, as we have shown elsewhere and following Zieher (2001), children's different food practices reflect different familial conceptualisations of their responsibilities and participation, as children, within everyday family life, conceptualisations that turn out not to be class-based to any great extent (James *et al.* 2009). Instead, they are more firmly explicable in terms of different conceptualisations of child–adult relations between families. These range from those families that are traditionally hierarchical to those in which children's independence and agency are fostered and facilitated. Here, therefore, we do not address social class as an analytical concept for understanding children's food practices but instead focus on the ways in which ideas of generation shape the food relationships between children and adults within the family.

Therefore, we first consider what 'snacking', as it is constructed in family narratives as a specific eating practice of *children*, reveals about the nature of family life and the constitution of child–adult relations within the family. Second, we broaden the discussion to consider how food moralities – and indeed immoralities – are negotiated in relation to the different food consumption practices of child and adult family members. But in so doing we are not proposing a hierarchy of good and bad foods, or suggesting that such values are rooted, necessarily or inherently, in specific foodstuffs. Rather, what we demonstrate is that these food moralities are subject to ongoing familial negotiations and that, although they may often be contextualised by wider populist notions of food morality, their most significant import lies elsewhere: food moralities are generationally nuanced, serving to mediate child–adult relations within particular cultural contexts that are informed by local cultural practices. Thus, we suggest, child–adult relations are discursively constructed through the creation, contestation and recreation of particular food narratives and – what is most significant – through specific moralities imposed upon children's, rather than adults', eating practices. Following the work of Morgan (1996) we argue, therefore, that such emergent food moralities are fundamental to 'doing' family, serving to promote a shared understanding of the generational values and practices which carry meanings associated with 'family' and which give rise to particular subject positions both for children and their parents.

Methods

The data that this discussion draws upon were generated through the *Children as Family Participants* study[5] which explored children's participation in the everyday practice of family life. Focusing on food and eating practices in and across different forms of family and different family styles, the project looked at children's experiences and perceptions of their contributions to the family through the everyday negotiations that take place with parents and other family members around food.

Following University Research Ethics approval, children aged between 11 and 12 were recruited from year groups in four schools in the North Midlands and South Yorkshire (UK). Three of the schools were located in urban areas: an inner city school in an area of significant social deprivation; a multi-ethnic inner city school and; a school located in an affluent, suburban area. The fourth school was located in a rural area with a wide geographical catchment. Consent was obtained from 108 children and their parents to participate in the first phase of data collection (54 girls and 54 boys) in which semi-structured interviews were carried out in small friendship groups, usually consisting of two children, during the school day. Children described themselves as having a range of ethnic identities, however the majority described themselves as 'white British'.

A second, later phase of data collection was also undertaken. A sub-sample of children was selected to represent a diversity of (overlapping) family forms: single parent families; families with only one child; families with two or more children; and families following a restricted diet due to health, religious or social reasons. Thirty children agreed to take part in a second interview (18 girls and 12 boys) which was carried out in the family home of each child. One parent from each family[6] also participated: parental and child interviews were carried out separately.[7]

Children's snacks and other food practices

In their discussions of children's snacking practices, both the adults and children that we interviewed made reference to eating a wide variety of snack food items such as crisps, yoghurts, toast/bread and jam, toasties, crackers and cereals. None of these foods are, of course, consumed exclusively by children and, indeed, our data show that adults as well as children acknowledge a liking for and the consumption of such snack foods. And yet, interestingly, in our data, it is only *children's* snacking behaviour involving such food items that draws particular comment in both children's own narratives and in those of their parents. This provides a first indication of the way in which generation serves as a distinctive marker in the negotiation of familial food practices and moralities.

A second more substantive clue can be seen, however, in the ways in which, within families, parents' own consumption of such foodstuffs is actively differentiated from the snacking choices and food behaviours of their children. This is achieved by distinguishing between children's snacks, and children's food more broadly, in terms of its quality. Again these distinctions appear in both parents' and children's narratives, thereby revealing a shared familial understanding of these constructions. Brian, for example, describes his dad's yoghurts as 'special yoghurts which has custard and fruit in them'. Children's snacks, by contrast, are more mundane or of lower quality. As George notes, his mother 'doesn't get us the nice biscuits. She gets the mud biscuits as we call them. The biscuits that don't taste very nice so we don't eat them'. Thus, the distinction between children's and adults' food is made within families, in part, in terms of food quality and, by implication, morality: the better the quality of the food, the greater its moral value, a hierarchical classification that mirrors the hierarchy of child–adult relations that is commonplace in many families.

This differentiation of children's snacks and food from that of adults' is, however, further reinforced through adult-imposed constraints on access to particular foodstuffs. That the custard and fruit yogurts are destined only for his Dad is clear from what Brian goes on to say: 'And he tells us never, ever to touch them yoghurts. If you touch them yoghurt and he's gonna come back and spoon and eat us'. Similarly, in a joint interview, Owen's parents acknowledge that they buy 'chocolate rations' for themselves and although they do not hide these from the children, laughingly, they admit that they 'make it quite clear [to the children] they can't have them'. Other parents did describe hiding 'adult' snacks from their children: Harry's mother buys 'good biscuits, good cakes' for adult consumption only, which are subsequently hidden from the children. In other families, such adult foods are stored in places that are difficult for children to access, as Tom makes clear when he refers to the 'top cupboard' in his house.

> We do have this top cupboard which has got like nice sweet things in. Maybe some crisps and chocolate but they may be for special occasions or something. But like it's not only for the grown-ups but only the grown-ups can go and eat. Like get, bring it down or, we'd have to ask permission.

These micro-geographies are therefore both constitutive of the distinction between children's and adults' foods and eating practices and of the different statuses of child and adult within the family. Thus, when one mother, Laura, admits to eating the same snacks as her children, she adds that she should have been 'a bit more sneaky' to avoid her children noticing. Being caught eating 'children's snacks' threatens not only to undermine the construction of such foodstuffs *as* children's food but also, by implication, the generational difference and separateness that constitutes an important index of adult–child relations within families (Cook 2009).

Laura's recognition of her need to be 'a bit more sneaky' is also instructive, however, about the ongoing construction and negotiation of child–parent relations within families that is apparent elsewhere in our data. For example, children themselves recognise and reflect on the distinction made between children's and adults' snacks and are active in contesting the latter's availability. Mandy describes 'stealing' sweets that were hidden in the 'top cupboard' while, in the following extract, Erin demonstrates an understanding of the complexity of the generational food rules within her family as she seeks to negotiate access to her mother's forbidden, 'adult' food:

> ... my favourite chocolate's 'Bourneville' and she's got a big bar of it in the fridge which is really annoying so every now and then I can like I'll say, 'I've just had a piece of fruit or yoghurt, please can I have a bit of chocolate?

Thus, it is in the familial designation of certain foodstuffs as belonging to children, rather than adults (and vice versa), that particular bars of chocolate or particular biscuits come to play an integral part in the construction and reconstruction of personal and generational relationships within families (Smart 2007).

However, both adults and children differentiate children's food from that of adults not just in terms of its quality or restricted access. Children's food practices are marginalised, by both children and adults, as lesser eating practices than those concerned with the real and proper business of family eating. This process of marginalisation is acknowledged by parents and children, for example, in their discussion of special occasions involving food, such as birthday parties or other forms of celebration. During such out-of-the-ordinary occasions, children can be allowed snacks and other foodstuffs that are normally restricted or prohibited as part of family eating, as Gail's mother describes;

> Coke. It would be a treat. So if it was a birthday party or if we've had, like we had a party this weekend [ ] And if we go out to the pub they [the children] will have 'Coke'... (pause) but they know that I wouldn't normally buy it. Or Christmas time I buy it.

69

Thus, by emphasising their availability, to children, only on special occasions or as treats, foods such as pizza, ice cream and carbonated drinks are clearly marked as extra-ordinary and as different from proper, family food and usual (normal) family practices (Johansson *et al.* 2009).

Similarly, children's eating with their friends is not family eating and children may therefore, on these occasions, also be allowed to eat differently, as Joel illustrates:

Joel ... if I have a friend round we'll have like burgers and chips and stuff like that.

Interviewer: Yeah. And wouldn't you have that if you didn't have a friend round?

Joel Well, I would sometimes but normally I wun't.

Interviewer: Yeah. And where do you eat then when your friends are round?

Joel Er, *(pause)* in the living room.

Interviewer: Do you?

Joel Yeah.

Interviewer: And does your Mum eat with you or not?

Joel Not normally.

The different eating practices that are permitted and enabled at such times are also acknowledged by parents. When her daughter's friends come for tea, Cara's mother tends to 'give food what kids like. Pizza, things like that, fish and chips or wedges and chips, smileys'. Even those parents who usually restrict such processed food make exceptions when friends are visiting. On these occasions they were prepared to provide what they refer to as 'child friendly food', as Ian's mother illustrates:

I tend to like we've got a little boy coming tomorrow and I tend to do more children friendly food when somebody's coming over. But the rest of the time we tend to eat more sort of adult type meals but if there's a friend coming over then I will try and make it a bit more child friendly... kind of like sausages... maybe pizza or something if somebody's coming over really whereas we don't tend, we, we tend to eat more sort of like pasta bakes and lasagne and stuff like that. Or chillis and stuff if it's. But I wouldn't, I'd, it would depend on the child really but it would be more child friendly food if we were having somebody over... I would be a lot more patient about that [ ] I wouldn't impose like I would make my kids do.

Thus, the generational marginalisation of children's food from mainstream 'proper' food is achieved within families both through the type and quality of food that is designated as 'children's food', the restrictions placed upon access and also its out of family-time patterns of consumption. This process of marginalisation can be seen most clearly in parents' relaxed attitudes towards children's food consumption in the time immediately following the end of the school day: the temporal organisation of the school day means that many children in secondary schools (as the 11–12 year olds interviewed for this study were) return home while their parents are still out at work. They therefore experience this period of time in the home as non-family time and as a time when they are permitted to consume children's food. As Brian's mother recognises, they 'come home, (and) it's straight for the (snack) drawer'. The challenge that this practice might otherwise represent to 'proper' family food is rationalised by Gwen's mother in the following manner: she comments that her daughter will 'have to have a snack after school, there's no way she can manage'. Following Prout (2000), this construction of children's bodies as capricious, wilful and demanding thus allows 'children's snacking', which as we discuss in more detail below is often seen by parents as morally problematic, to be safely accommodated. In these ways, then, the challenges to proper food that such 'snacking' might represent is minimised and the potential disruption to family eating routines that it might otherwise present is further offset by many families setting time-limits on such free snacking practices. Children can 'snack' when they come in from school but not in the hour or so preceding the family meal.

Children's snacking, and their food and eating practices more generally, are therefore 'othered' in relation to the consumption of 'proper' food and proper family meals. Furthermore, as we have already suggested, such food and eating practices are also constituted as morally different since they lie outside cultural constructions of 'proper' family food – the food that matters both in terms of nutrition and in terms of family eating. In the next section, therefore, we consider how food moralities – the distinctions between proper and improper, good and bad food and eating practices – are negotiated and maintained within families and, in particular, how children's consumption of 'children's food' is conceptually – and practically – managed by parents whose job it is to uphold familial standards in relation to food practices.

Family food moralities

Many of the foodstuffs referred to by children and parents as 'children's snacks' treats and, more generally, 'children's food' can be readily characterised as just the sort of foods that the NHS Change for Life campaign warns about; they are high in sugar, fat, calories and salt, foods that 'we shouldn't eat too much' (see footnote 2). Chocolate, sweets, biscuits, cakes and some (bought) savoury products such as sausage rolls, are referred to as 'children's snacks' by children and adults alike, despite the fact that adults sometime eat them too. And significantly such foodstuffs were widely characterised by both children and adults as bad food. The problematic connotations of such foods (often referred to as 'junk' foods) means that they are subject to explicit value judgements: 11-year-old Mary, for example, commented that 'when I know like that I've been eating just like junk food most, most of the time, I think I've done something wrong'. This self-critical observation raises questions, however, about the extent to which children themselves, like Mary, share such negative understandings of the kinds of food they themselves often choose to eat and whether they are active in negotiating these meanings through the day-to-day interactions that take place within families. In this section, therefore we consider the ways in which wider cultural moralities about food intersect with the familial understandings of proper and improper food and generational relations outlined above.

First, it is clear that children draw upon a variety of discourses in their food-related narratives. In the rural school, for example, the notion of good food was constructed by some children in terms of food 'as it should be'. While food-as-it-should be could be organic food (Tom: 'generally organic foods are more flavoursome and stuff'), it was more generally understood by these children to be food that had not been interfered with. Food-as-it-should-be was therefore characterised as food that is largely free of additives and colourants, not overly processed or sweetened. Alicia compares 'food-as-it should-be' with food 'out of a packet':

> ... if someone puts something in front of me then 'cause by looking at it you can tell. If it's out of a packet or if it's like (pause) just not (pause) right and [ ] well you can, you can tell like if it's like mass production can't you because there's like everything always looks the same. But like say (pause) say I made a milkshake yeah?

> And, and [ ] you got one from the shop and just put 'em both in a cup you can tell which one's better for you because it's not got all the colourings in and all the 'e numbers' and stuff.

And that in a separate interview, Alicia's mother makes similar comments, attests to a shared family understanding that valorises this kind of food:

> ... you know (there are) certain things to avoid and. Well you just know if it looks a funny colour and it's got loads of packaging on then it can't really be good for you.

Similarly, Brian avoids one particular orange flavoured drink, 'because of the amount of sugar content' and Brian's mother concurs:

> You're buying something that you think is orange juice and then [ ] 'cause it was very sugary wasn't it. 'Right, no more'.

In a shared family narrative, this drink is constructed as an exemplar of a 'bad' foodstuff and contrasted with food 'as it should be', this suggests, therefore, that within these rural families there is some commonality of understanding about food moralities, which may reflect local cultural practices. Both parents and children share a familial understanding of what proper food is and should be.

These discourses about the positive benefits of organic and unadulterated food were, however, minority ones and were not reflected in the narratives of other children or parents living in more urban settings. Yet, although their frames of reference were different, parents and children in these other families similarly shared understandings around good and bad food. In this instance these were influenced, overwhelmingly, by media representations of unhealthy and 'bad' foods, as George's mother made clear when describing how she makes judgements about food:

> Well it's usually through the TV to be perfectly honest. Yeah. You know, there's always something that pops up in these programmes and food programmes. [ ] Just on all the things that do come up that are really bad [ ] And there are a lot of things that are said to be healthy that aren't really. Things like the, I mean, we were, we were taking the 'Actimels'.[8] And it came out that there were six spoons of sugar in each one.

Both children and their parents made reference to a variety of contemporary UK television food and lifestyle programmes, often by reference to the celebrity who fronted these – Jamie Oliver, Gillian McKeith, Paul McKenna – and also, explicitly by name to 'School Dinners', 'You are what you eat', 'Honey we're killing the kids' and 'Supersize me'. During data collection, in 2006 and 2007, there was widespread awareness among children and their parents of 'that Jamie thing': even amongst children who had not actually watched the specific television programmes.[9] Tess, for example, told us about some older boys in her school who had watched Jamie Oliver making chicken nuggets:

> ... and even Dominic says it's disgusting 'cause, like, he's just chucking beans and peas all together and mushing it up. [ ] They said it was horrible. They said what we was eating wasn't chicken. It was some kind of thing what he'd, people are just making to look like chicken and taste like chicken when he wrapped it in some, some sort of skin. He'd made 'em chicken nuggets and it were disgusting. [ ] Well, I, erm, I, I've never had a chicken burger in my life after that day (laugh).

Ewan also discussed how chicken nuggets were made with his friend, asking:

> What did you think to that when they showed them what was in the chicken nuggets when they put it in the whisk? Put me off chicken nuggets. And I liked chicken nuggets back then. Not any more. Well, it showed children what were, what they were actually eating, what was actually in the fast food that they were eating.

> (Interviewer: So, do you think maybe kids don't know what's in food?)

> Ewan: I think they should do that. Yeah. I think they should do that here. Just like get a pile of, just lob it in. Like, put it into a chicken nugget, just like put it into a pot (laughing) just like gooey. [ ] So, like, all the percentage, blub and e-numbers, blub, blub

Parents too reacted to revelations about chicken nuggets with surprise and horror. Isla's mother, for example, describes them as 'disgusting' and herself as 'appalled at the diet that I saw, or the stuff that went in'. In her work on the feeding of babies and young children, Murphy (2003, p. 455) notes that feeding choices within families 'are made in the context of a powerful medicalised scientific discourse about how children ought to be fed'. And, as consumers of programmes such as School Dinners, our data show that children and their parents interact directly with such medicalised discourses as Brian illustrates when he comments that these programmes are 'really like saving their lives, 'cause salt overtakes and stuff like that'.

Thus, children's and parent's awareness of what one child summarised as the 'Jamie thing', serves to reflect and reinforce the problematisation of 'children's food' which, as we suggested earlier, is already marginalised in a variety of other ways in everyday family practices. And since parents who do not control their children's access to 'bad' food and who support eating practices that are contrary to expert advice raise questions about the legitimacy of their parenting practices and run the risk of being seen as bad parents (Coveney 2000, Murphy 2000), many parents sought to further control and restrict their children's access to 'bad' food. Owen's mother, for example, stopped buying some foods,

'cause he, if there's anything in the fridge like that like sausage rolls or crisps in the cupboard that's what he'll (her son) go for.

Such prohibited foods were frequently characterised in terms of specific branded products or particular food types. As Jack said, bad food is 'some sort of chips and [ ] when it's the all the fat things like pizzas' (Jack): ironically, these are just the foods that, as we showed earlier, both children and adults class as 'children's food'. It is this paradox that we next address.

Managing food moralities within the family

We have argued so far that 'children's food' does not form part of proper family dinners, and that within the food moralities of both children and adults, it represents marginalised and improper kinds of food stuffs. Occupying the lower rungs of the contemporary moral hierarchy of food, it neatly resonates however with children's often subordinate position within the generational hierarchy of family life. But given that, over recent years, such food has been subject to considerable media attention, as noted above, and has been characterised as problematic in healthy eating discourses, this creates a paradox for families: how should children's consumption of such 'children's foods' be managed in everyday family life if, core to the construction of good parenting is the assumption that, as vulnerable subjects, children need protection from such bad foods which they seem unable to resist on their own. As Jack's mother claims, her son's preference would be for 'all the junk food you could think'.

Parents are not alone in recognising this paradox. Children's narratives can also reflect this idea: when asked whether she felt that schools should introduce healthy foods, Eleanor replied that 'If kids choose they could, they could pick the wrong things'. Amy too highlights children's assumed vulnerability, suggesting that her sister could not be trusted to make 'good' food choice without adult intervention: Amy comments that their mother will 'like say you've got to eat ten carrots or whatever and then I'll make you something else. Because otherwise she'll have, my sister'd just eat fish fingers all the time, or chocolate'.

As Christensen has noted children's vulnerability is 'a construction of the way in which children perceive themselves and are perceived by others. It is embedded in cultural understandings of the child as a social person, of the child's body and conceptions of health and illness' (Christensen 2000, p. 57). However, unsurprisingly, while sharing the food moralities of their parents, children also act in tension with this construction of vulnerability by resisting parental constraints on their consumption of 'bad' food and negotiating alternate ways to act in relation to family. George, for example, was not allowed to eat a particular type of sweets at home as his mother was concerned that they caused hyperactivity, but this did not stop him from buying them for himself outside of the home:

Honestly my Mum thinks we're still hyper on them. But when I went to the, I go down to the shops sometimes and I buy some sweets. And I used to have 'Skittles' 'cause they had 'em in the stand. And I got, I got them. And I told all my friends that I would go hyper and things. And they all prepared themselves. And then I ate them and I was fine. But my Mum still thinks we go hyper.

In reality, however, there were few parents who sought – or expected to be able to – exert complete control over their child's eating (see also Cook 2009). Indeed, for many parents, their food-related narratives evidence their recognition and acceptance of children's agency, albeit that such expressions are often managed, within the family (as we have discussed earlier), through the marginalisation of children's practices. George's mother, for example, remarks ruefully that when her children are hungry between proper meals, 'They just tend to have fruit and usually have a tin of biscuits when we're not looking'.

This reference to fruit eating is of particular interest since it is a management strategy that also draws upon powerful external moral discourses of food. If chicken nuggets have become a metonym for 'bad' food, fruit has become a metonym for 'good' food and is key to the generational negotiations around food consumption that take place between children and their parents. Parents try, for example, to off-set the negative effects for their children of their consumption of 'bad' food by insisting that children eat fruit as well as, rather than instead of, junk food:

> I said: 'you're not having ice-cream unless you have a piece of fruit with it' ... and it's a battle to get them to do that ... if it was up to them they would have all ice-cream! (Jack's mother)

Thus, just as Erin had sought to negotiate access to forbidden adult food (her mother's bar of chocolate) by emphasising that she had 'just had a piece of fruit' (as described earlier), so other children also reflected this trade off, in their food-related negotiations with their parents. As Dan notes, 'Well, if I've just had a big bowl of fruit or something... I ask for a, like a Kit Kat or something'. Within the generational frame of family life children are therefore active in the ongoing negotiation of family food moralities and, when they have played the game – eaten the fruit – if parents still seek to prevent them from eating what they want, children feel more able to go behind their parents' backs to access restricted 'children's food', as Brian makes clear when he confides that 'sometimes I'd just nick, kinda like a quick little chocolate bar just like one of these little niblets that we have [ ] kind of like just a little finger biscuit you know like one of them mini KitKat things'.

Conclusion: the construction of children's food and eating practices in everyday family life

While 'snacking' provides an introduction to the consideration of how children's and adult's eating practices are differentiated within families, we have argued that snacking is but one, albeit noteworthy, manifestation of children's food and children's eating practices as they are constructed within family discourses. Their construction, as *children's* practices in family narratives is informative, offering, as we have suggested, insights into the nature of family life and the constitution of child–adult relations: the differentiation between children's and adults' food and food practices that was evident in our data, both reflects and is constitutive of generational difference and separateness within families (Cook 2009).

As Alanen (2001) points out, generation is a relational concept which is constructed on an ongoing, recurrent basis through the complex set of day-to-day practices through which 'people become (are constructed as) "children" while other people become (are constructed as) "adults"' (Alanen 2001, pp. 20–21). Furthermore, as Alanen (2001) goes on to note, focusing upon relational, generational processes highlights the significance of children's (as well as adults') agency: 'the "powers" (or lack of them), of those positioned as children, to influence, organize, coordinate and control events taking place in their everyday world's' (Alanen 2001, p. 21). As we have shown, in the construction of children's food and eating practices children's agency is both enabled within families, allowing children to exercise a degree of choice over the food they eat, and constrained, through the reification of hierarchical generational relationships within the family.

However, while the construction of children's food and children's food practices – and thus child–adult relations – is both a practical and a material process as Alanen suggests and as we have also shown, the construction of children's food practices, and thus of child–adult relations, is *also* explicitly a moral process. Children's food is subject, in our data, to explicit value judgements and widely characterised by both children and adults, as bad food. Furthermore, children's eating practices are marginalised in out-of-family-time and 'othered' in relation to the important business of 'proper' family meals. If the significance of practices derives 'from their location in wider systems of meaning' (Morgan 1996, p. 190), how adults' and children's lives intersect with broader cultural messages around food and eating is, as we have argued, fundamental to the ongoing negotiation of generationally nuanced food moralities within the family. Thus we have demonstrated how understandings of good and bad food within families are influenced by local cultural practices and by broader cultural understandings communicated, in particular, through media representations.

We began by remarking upon media coverage illustrating contemporary concern for children's food and eating practices. We have shown, however, that despite this moral panic, familial constructions of children's snacking and their other food and eating practices are managed within the ebb and flow of everyday family lives so that, rather than negating the importance of family food and togetherness, they become 'constitutive of [the] inter-generational relations and generational identities' (Curtis *et al.* 2009, p. 92) through which the idea of 'family' is itself constructed on an ongoing and everyday basis.

Notes

1. http://www.dailymail.co.uk/news/article-408812/British-children-eat-825-snacks-year.html
2. http://www.nhs.uk/change4life/
3. http://www.nhs.uk/change4life/Pages/MakeChangeSnackCheck.aspx
4. http://familyrelationships.org.uk/the-importance-of-families-eating-together
5. The *Children as Family Participants* study formed part of an interdisciplinary Research Programme, *Changing Families, Changing Food*, funded by the Leverhulme Trust (http://www.shef.ac.uk/familiesandfood/)
6. On occasions, however, both parents chose to take part and were interviewed.
7. All children have been assigned pseudonyms: parents were not assigned separate pseudonyms and extracts from their transcripts are referred to as the 'parent of ...'.
8. Actimel is a trademarked 'probiotic drinking yogurt' which is marketed as having the potential to ' help support your body's defences' (http://www.actimel.co.uk/About/Default.aspx Accessed 8 August 2009)
9. Jamie Oliver has hosted a number of food related television programmes: '*Jamies School Dinners*', in which the celebrity chef campaigned to ban 'junk' food in children's school dinners was particularly influential at the time of data collection. http://www.channel4.com/life/microsites/J/jamies_school_dinners/

References

Alanen, L., 2001. Explorations in generational analysis. *In*: L. Alanen and B. Mayall, eds. *Conceptualising adult–child relations*. London: Routledge-Falmer, 11–22.

Bell, D. and Valentine, G., 2003. *Consuming geographies: we are what we eat*. London: Routledge.

Blake, M., Mellor, J., Crane, L., and Osz, B., 2009. Eating in time, eating up time. *In*: P. Jackson, ed. *Changing families, changing food*. London: Palgrave Macmillan, 187–204.

Brembeck, H., 2005. Home to McDonald's: upholding the family dinner with the help of McDonald's. *Food, Culture and Society*, 8 (2), 215–226.

Charles, N. and Kerr, M., 1988. *Women, food and families*. Manchester: Manchester University Press.

Christensen, P., 2000. Childhood and the cultural constitution of vulnerable bodies. *In*: A. Prout ed, ed. *The body, childhood and society*. London: Macmillan Press, 38–59.

Cook, D.T., 2009. Children's subjectivities and commercial meaning: the delicate battle mothers wage when feeding their children. *In*: A. James, A. Kjorholt and V. Tingstad, eds. *Children, food and identity in everyday life*. Basingstoke: Palgrave, 112–129.

Coveney, J., 2000. *Food, morals, and meaning. The pleasure and anxiety of eating*. London: Routledge.

Crawford, D. and Jeffery, R., eds., 2005. *Obesity prevention and public health*. Oxford: Oxford University Press.

Curtis, P., James, A., and Ellis, K., 2009. 'She's got a really good attitude to healthy food... Nannan's drilled it into her': intergenerational relations within families. *In*: P. Jackson, ed. *Changing Families, Changing Food*. London: Palgrave Macmillan, 77–92.

Devault, M.L., 1994. *Feeding the family: the social organization of care as gendered work*. Chicago, IL: University of Chicago Press.

Gillis, J., 1996. Making time for family: the invention of family time(s) and the reinvention of family history. *Journal of Family History*, 21 (4), 4–21.

Green, T., Owen, J., Curtis, P., Smith, G., Ward, P., and Fisher, P., 2009. Making healthy families? *In*: P. Jackson, ed. *Changing families, changing food*. London: Palgrave Macmillan, 205–225.

Jackson, P., 2009. Introduction: food a lens on family life. *In*: P. Jackson, ed. *Changing families, changing food*. London: Palgrave Macmillan, 1–16.

Jackson, P., Olive, S., and Smith, G., 2009. Myths of the family meal: re-reading Edwardian life-histories. *In*: P. Jackson, ed. *Changing families, changing food*. London: Palgrave Macmillan, 131–145.

James, A., Curtis, P., and Ellis, K., 2009. Negotiating family, negotiating food: children as family participants? *In*: A. James, A. Kjorholt and V. Tingstad, eds. *Children, food and identity in everyday life*. Basingstoke: Palgrave Macmillan, 35–51.

Johansson, B., Mäkelä, J., Roos, G., Hillén, S., Hansen, G., Jensen, T., and Huotilainen, A., 2009. Nordic children's foodscapes: images and reflections. *Food, Culture and Society*, 12 (1), 25–51.

Lupton, D., 1996. *Food, the body and self*. London: Sage.

Morgan, D., 1996. *Family connections*. Cambridge: Polity Press.

Murcott, A., 1983. Cooking and the cooked: a note on the domestic preparation of meals. *In*: A. Murcott, ed. *The sociology of food and eating: essays on the sociological significance of food*. Aldershot: Gower.

Murphy, E., 2003. Expertise and forms of knowledge in the government of families. *The Sociological Review*, 51 (4), 433–462.

Prout, A., ed., 2000. *The body, childhood and society*. London: MacMillan.

Shaw, A., McMunn, A., and Field, J., 2000. *The Scottish health survey 1998*. London: Joint Health Surveys Unit.

Silva, E.B. and Smart, C., 2004. *The new family?* London: Sage.

Smart, C., 2007. *Personal life*. Cambridge: Polity.

Sproston, K. and Primatesta, P., eds., 2003. *Health survey for England 2003: risk factors for cardiovascular disease*. London: TSO.

Willets, A., 1997. Bacon sandwiches got the better of me' Meat-eating and vegetarianism in South-East London. *In*: P. Caplan, ed. *Food, health, and identity*. London: Routledge, 111–130.

Wills, W., Backett-Milburn, K., Gregory, S., and Lawton, J., 2008. 'If the food looks dodgy I dinnae eat it': teenagers' accounts of food and eating practices in socio-economically disadvantaged families. *Sociological Research Online*, 13), 1–2. (http://www.socresonline.org.uk/13/1/15.html)

Zieher, H., 2001. Dependent, independent and interdependent relations: children as members of the family household in West Berl. *In*: L. Alanen and B. Mayall, eds. *Conceptualizing child–adult relations*. London: Routledge Falmer, 37–53.

Food and family practices: teenagers, eating and domestic life in differing socio-economic circumstances

Kathryn Backett-Milburn[a], Wendy Wills[b], Mei-Li Roberts[c] and
Julia Lawton[a]

[a]*Public Health Sciences, School of Clinical Sciences and Community Health, College of Medicine and Veterinary Medicine, The University of Edinburgh, Medical School, Edinburgh, Scotland, UK, [b]CRIPACC, University of Hertfordshire, Hatfield, UK, [c]BACYS Degree Course Leader/Research Fellow, UHI Centre for Rural Childhood, Perth College UHI, Perth UK*

This paper draws on accounts from young teenagers and their parents in two linked qualitative studies of families living in Scotland in differing socio-economic circumstances. We compare and contrast teenager experiences of eating practices and food choice in these families. We show the range of meanings attached to how, where and what these teenagers and their parents described as everyday eating behaviours at home and locate these in the wider constraints, opportunities and aspirations affecting their lives.

Introduction

'Family' is created through a myriad of mundane everyday practices (Morgan 1996) of which domestic provision of food remains a central element. However, although families are accepted as the primary setting for the establishment of patterns of food choice and consumption in childhood (Dietz 2001), how parents and family background actually affect what teenagers eat at home on a daily basis is less clear. Not only is the collective identity of 'family' being created through everyday food choices and eating behaviours in the home but so also are the individual identities of family members (Devault 1991, Lupton 1994, Valentine 1999, Wright-St Clair *et al.* 2005).

We draw on two linked qualitative studies carried out in Scotland with young teenagers and their parents living in contrasting socio-economic circumstances. In study 1 we sampled those living in more disadvantaged socio-economic circumstances, more 'working class' (w/c) families, and in study 2 those living in higher SES, more 'middle class' (m/c) families. Here we examine the accounts of food and family practices of young teenagers in their homes and the negotiations between parents and teenagers surrounding these processes (Dixey *et al.*

2001, Kaufman and Karpati 2007). We relate these to the wider constraints, opportunities and aspirations affecting families' lives (Backett-Milburn *et al.* 2006, Devine *et al.* 2006).

An important focus of our work was on the question 'does class matter?' We draw on already published data from study 1 (w/c) and new analyses, some of which is under consideration for publication, from study 2 (m/c). Through making comparisons between these two sets of findings, we highlight issues of class-based dispositions and practices. We first show how the differing domestic environments and expectations of parents in each study may be seen as the background for the teenagers' own accounts. We then explore the teenagers' own perspectives on tastes, preferences and parental control.

Background

Food and eating related practices in the home are both embedded in and reflective of people's everyday family and domestic lives and socio-cultural circumstances; they are dynamic and culturally responsive (Crossley 2004, Warin *et al.* 2008). Family routines and identities are created and reinforced through the preparation of food for other family members (Caplan 1997, Mintz and DuBois 2002). Individuals become connected when they eat together (Wright-St Clair *et al.* 2005) although the sharing of food in families with young teenagers can highlight tensions and conflict during this phase of the life course when young people seek to become more autonomous.

Young people's diets have come increasingly under the spotlight as considerable attention has been paid to the so-called 'obesogenic environment' (Egger and Swinburn 1997), focussing particularly on the dietary, commercial, lifestyle and social contexts which appear to foster less healthy eating practices (Cunningham 2003, Colls and Evans 2008). Consequently, there is more information about the characteristics and contexts of population groups who seem particularly affected by health damaging circumstances and environments, and weight increasing behaviours, than about other, usually more affluent, groups who seem somewhat less affected by these trends (Ball and Crawford 2005). It is valuable also to understand the social and cultural conditions which might be seen as promoting more positive dietary health and physical wellbeing in the face of trends which seem to be challenging these aspects of teenagers' lives (Sarlio-Lahteenkorva 2007).

Here we take social class as being a hierarchical (and unequal) framework of relationships which arise from the social organisation of labour, education, wealth and income (Bradley 1996). It is widely accepted that the unequal material circumstances associated with class distinctions influence peoples' lives and health (Williams 1995) and there has been a revival of interest in class studies in geography (Dowling 2009). Through examination of the everyday lived experience of deprivation or affluence we can see how class might underpin growing inequalities in health. Bourdieu (1984), in his work on habitus, argued that social distinctions are maintained through the production and control of bodily practices, which are often mundane and taken-for-granted (Williams 1995). This implies that daily practices and beliefs surrounding diet, health and weight might provide a 'structuring structure' which, whilst serving to distinguish one class group from another, would be 'neither known nor chosen by [such groups]' (Williams 2003, p. 143). A lack of qualitative research specifically focussing on families, class and eating practices means that the mechanisms which might explain differences and similarities between different groups remain largely unexplored.

However, in the related field of health relevant behaviour, Bourdieu and others suggested that lower social class groups may have a more utilitarian attitude towards health, valuing bodies free from illness and capable of performing everyday activities (Bourdieu 1984, d'Houtard and Field 1984). The middle-classes, however, may be more likely to value enhanced wellbeing, rather than merely a functional absence of disease (d'Houtard and Field 1984, Blaxter 1990).

Quantitative explorations of the role of class in explaining young peoples' health-relevant behaviours suggests that structurally determined experiences may not be as influential as in previous generations (West and Sweeting 2004). Such issues are, however, likely to be complex and dynamic. Some evidence, for example, suggests that young people from working class backgrounds start following potentially problematic health trajectories earlier than their middle class peers whilst other work indicates that, as young teenagers start to move away from family influence, this may perhaps result in a 'blending' of peer groups from differing socio-economic circumstances (West and Sweeting 2004).

It is important to understand children and young people as social actors in their own right; this also involves exploring their voices concerning food and eating (Christensen and James 2000, Metcalfe *et al.* 2008, Pike 2008). As they become teenagers, many parents may be willing to renegotiate the rules and boundaries set for their children (Backett-Milburn and Harden 2004). Nevertheless, at home, particularly in the areas of family food practices, teenagers may only be able to contest or define their autonomy within the constraints of their parents' behaviours and wishes. Consequently, their everyday domestic and dietary worlds can only be fully made sense of by examining their social lives more generally, for example through also exploring the practices and beliefs of family, siblings and friends. (Eldridge and Murcott 2000, Eckert 2004).

Existing literature indicates that socio-economic status remains an important factor underpinning food provision in families. For instance, family income often influences diet (Dowler and Calvert 1995, Grieshaber 1997), with socio-economically disadvantaged families tending to eat less 'healthily' than middle class families (Shaw *et al.* 2000, Sproston and Primatesta 2003). However, the meanings attached to mundane practices of food preparation and eating at home are also intimately connected with family 'habitus', the unconscious logic of practice and rules of acceptable consumption which underpin everyday routines and behaviours (Warin *et al.* 2008). From this perspective, the most taken-for-granted aspects of preparing, eating and choosing food on a daily basis are based on accumulated habits and preferences built up within distinct social groups (Bourdieu 1984). In these ways, whether for the working class or middle class (Tomanovic 2004), shared past and present knowledge and experience of the social world continue to shape individuals' (and families') identities and understandings of what is appropriate and possible for 'people like me' (Reay 2004). Our two linked studies therefore aimed to tease out some of the ways in which class matters at home.

Description of studies and methods

Although designed and funded independently of each other, taken together these two studies were intended to explore the ways in which class might underpin perceptions and practices regarding teenagers' diet, health and weight. Study 2 (m/c) (Backett-Milburn *et al.* 2008) was designed to facilitate a critical examination of some of the key findings emerging from study 1 (w/c).[1] The linked studies therefore explored many similar themes and the topic guides were broadly comparable. Through interviews with teenagers and the parents/carers who were the main food providers, the two studies also aimed to revisit the relevance of theories about class-based predispositions and distinctions for everyday dietary practices in families.

In both studies an iterative qualitative approach was taken, allowing the exploration of themes emerging during data collection in addition to those formulated at the outset (Britten *et al.* 1995). In each study 36 young people aged 13–15 years were interviewed, as were 34 working class and 35 middle class parents/main food providers. The samples comprised equal numbers of boys and girls.

Following ethical approval from relevant education authorities, we gained access to several schools in first, relatively disadvantaged, and second, more advantaged areas in Eastern

Scotland. Schools were selected in part on the basis of the numbers of students eligible for free school meals (a proxy indicator in the UK for socio-economic status). For each study we made complex assessments of socio-economic status. A screening questionnaire was administered to collect young people's socio-demographic information (parent/s' occupation; home postcode; family affluence, household composition) and details of their physical activity and favourite or regularly consumed foods. For each study we also selected teenagers on the basis of at least one parent's occupation according to NS-SEC (Office of National Statistics 2005). Family affluence was ascertained from responses to two items adapted from the Family Affluence Scale (Currie *et al.* 1997) – whether the teenager had their own bedroom and if the family had at least one holiday in the past year. Deprivation was assessed using the 2001 Carstairs scores for Scottish postcode sectors (McClone 2004) and the Scottish Index of Deprivation.[2] The families interviewed were predominantly White/Scottish, reflecting the ethnicity of the local population. Double consent was sought for the teenagers: parents were asked to 'opt out' if they did not wish their child to participate; young people and parents each gave their own written consent to be interviewed.

For each study, interviews were conducted firstly with the teenagers, later with the parents who were identified by the teenagers as their main food provider (these were predominantly mothers, though several grandparents were interviewed as the guardian/main food provider in study 1 (w/c)). Qualitative interviews, lasting about one hour, took place in teenagers' homes and were tape recorded with their consent. The topic guide was similar for both studies and, each time, the parents' guides mirrored those used previously with the young people. We asked all interviewees to talk through typical and non-typical days enabling us to probe, in some detail, about all food consumed by the participating teenager and his/her family and the context for this consumption (where, with whom and when consumption took place). In this way food and eating were explored in the context of descriptions of the everyday lives of parents and teenagers at home, school, work and leisure.

Tapes were transcribed verbatim and anonymised. Throughout the analysis, selected transcripts were read by each team member, along with the research fellow's field notes and interview summaries. Emerging themes were noted independently. Regular analytical team meetings were held to discuss recurrent themes and any accounts that did not fit with the emerging thematic framework (Boyatzis 1998). The analysis proceeded until the team felt that each broad theme had been fully considered and defined, with continuous reference to the original transcripts. Some of the insights gained in study 2 (m/c) developed iteratively through comparisons with study 1 (w/c). Analysis focused on each broad theme that had emerged, with each team member independently considering finer, sub-themes. These were discussed as a team until consensus was reached. QSR NUD*IST was used for data coding and retrieval. Any names used in quotations here are pseudonyms.

Findings

Parental perspectives on managing young teenagers' food practices at home

We begin with the parents' perspectives to show some of the background framing the teenagers' accounts. In both studies, teenagers reported instances of parental control of their food choices at home through rules, expectations or 'standards' of food and eating practices. Although young peoples' accounts suggested they could also negotiate some flexibility around meal time patterns, few interviewees in either study reported trying to bend parental food rules or change parental food provisioning practices to any great degree. The working class and middle class parents' perspectives on managing young teenagers' food practices at home were, however, somewhat different. It is important that these are understood as embedded in the broader habitus and socio-economic circumstances/environments in which these families lived. Working class and middle class parents' perspectives will now be discussed in turn and comparisons returned to in the conclusions.

One major difference between the two studies was in the amount of control parents seemed to feel they should, or indeed could, exercise over teenagers' food consumption at home. In study 1 (w/c) the working class interviewees appeared largely to accept that, within the economic constraints affecting the kinds of foods provided at home, their young teenagers could make their own dietary choices. It was also evident in the working class study that, even though commensality might be valued, many of these teenagers were able regularly to eat elsewhere in the house, or on their own, for example in their rooms or in front of the television. Reflecting findings from other studies, it appeared to be the exception rather than the rule for times, places and contents of meals or snacks to coincide for the working class teenagers and their parents on any kind of regular basis (Eldridge and Murcott 2000). For instance, in about half of the working class families it was reported that teenagers always, or nearly always, ate at the same time, and in the same room, as the rest of their family (not all of this sample owned or used a table which could accommodate all family members); in the middle class sample almost all of the families reported commensality round a table to be the norm in their homes.

In study 1 (w/c), many parents spoke about their young teenagers' food choices and eating practices as being increasingly their own responsibility. Many of these parents said things such as 'at his age he'll eat what he wants to eat' (Alec's mother) and 'I just leave him up to hisself' (Neil's mother). One mother spoke about her difficulties in exercising control over her daughter's eating as follows:

> I think for me, it's important for her going to school with even a bowl of cereal or a piece of fruit or something like that. But her appearance is more important and she'll maybe grab a packet of crisps going up the road, which is not, in my view it's not, it's no good enough, but what can I do? I mean I cannae (cannot) force food down her neck. (Leanne's mother) (Backett-Milburn *et al.* 2006)

The working class parents seemed also to feel that their teenagers had strong food preferences and tastes, which should be accommodated; they described in detail what each of their children liked and disliked to eat. They seldom seemed to insist that teenagers should eat anything they disliked even if, as was particularly the case with vegetables and sometimes fruit, the majority of our working class parents also clearly stated that they saw these as being 'good for them'. Despite the fact that almost all of these parents said that healthy eating was important, most tended not to question their teenager's distaste for many 'healthier' foodstuffs, though they did say that they tried to counteract this with some of the food provided at home. Having relatively limited food budgets also seemed to affect parents' behaviour; it seemed important to them that food was not wasted and was also fairly shared within the family. In this regard, for instance, some parents who described their offspring as 'good eaters' said this not because the teenager ate 'healthy' foods but because s/he did not complain about or ate all of the food provided at home. Parents did, however, complain about the teenager if s/he took more than his/her allocated share, or another family member's share, of the foods they had bought for the home (Backett-Milburn *et al.* 2006).

These findings must be located in an appreciation of what is happening in many homes in the twenty-first century and the wider challenges facing families. Importantly, study 1 (w/c) also showed that their teenagers' eating behaviours were not the most pressing concerns expressed by this predominantly low income sample. Food choices and eating practices seemed to be given a fairly low priority in the 'hierarchy of worries' (Backett-Milburn *et al.* 2006) about 'risky' early teenage health-relevant and social behaviours. However, it was not that dietary matters were unimportant to these working class parents, they were simply viewed as less important than other worries about children at this particular age. Echoing other studies (Seaman *et al.*

2006), many of these less advantaged parents described the challenges and risks, such as poor school performance and opportunities, drugs, 'getting in with a bad crowd', facing their off-spring in their local environments both now and in the future. Such worries about teenagers and their futures may be exacerbated when parents are living in disadvantaged circumstances, have fewer resources at their disposal, and are raising their children in potentially less safe environments (Backett-Milburn *et al.* 2006).

Moving on now to study 2 (m/c) (Backett-Milburn *et al.* in press), like their more disadvantaged counterparts, the middle class parents spoke of wanting to provide good food at home and saw 'junk foods' as temptations for all teenagers. However, their interviews in study 2 (m/c) revealed a somewhat different environment and habitus in which they strove to achieve these aims. Importantly, most middle class parents' accounts appeared rooted in a taken-for-granted-ness that family members enjoyed good health (many did not in the more disadvantaged families). They described living in relatively secure and unthreatening environments regarding health and resources, and their children's experiences with school, friends and peers were largely experienced as positive. All family members, but there was a particularly strong focus on the children, were portrayed as able to lead active lives and afford to participate, for example, in organised sports, dance, gyms, music, etc., which were accorded strong social value. Although often admitting to falling short of their ideals, many middle class parents in this second study also spoke about trying to set a good example to their children with regard to health, eating well and leading what they described as full and active lives. By contrast, many of the working class parents seemed less secure about the example they might be setting in this regard.

These middle class parents' interviews showed they were also assuming continuing success and happiness for their children and, in this, they might be characterised as having future oriented 'hierarchies of luxury and choice'. Controlling and moulding teenagers' food practices, tastes and manners, particularly at home, were accorded high priority as the future social adult would need to accommodate various environments, including eating environments (Backett-Milburn *et al.* in press). Eating together as a family was one of the food practice ideals expressed by these middle class families. However, it appeared that, in practice, the number of children's after school activities often meant this was only achieved for some family members on any particular evening (though sitting together at table was still maintained). The parents also said that, on the whole, home cooked (or at least home-prepared) meals were provided most evenings; they aimed to cook from scratch as much as possible; and special efforts were made at weekends to offer more elaborate meals, such as roast dinners. The majority of middle class parents also described controlling portion sizes by serving food onto the plates for their families and/or telling their teenager if they felt they were eating too much or not taking enough vegetables. It seemed, from most middle class parents' interviews, that they thought their teenager was eating enough fruit and vegetables, even if they had to hide these in soups or stews, or the teenagers did not always enjoy them (Judith's mother: 'we eat – lots of vegetables, much to their horror'). These claims were borne out in the teenagers' own interviews.

However, as in the working class study, the free exercise of food choices and tastes in their children was felt by the middle class parents to become more of a challenge as they became teenagers. As Catriona's mother explained:

> I think you've got a role as a parent to guide them in what you think they should eat and to be honest with them but there's only... but teenagers have got independent minds and I think there's only so far you can go. (Backett-Milburn *et al.* in press)

Although controlling teenagers' eating practices was presented as an ongoing challenge by middle class parents, active supervision and surveillance of their diets was described, as was guiding tastes in 'the right direction'. This sense of overall parental control also permeated accounts of the other eating opportunities at home in the middle class study. In contrast to study 1 (w/c), the majority of middle class parents claimed either that the teenagers rarely took snacks without parental consent, stating that they had 'trained them well' (Nathan's mother), or that the teenager had sufficient self discipline to limit his/her own consumption of snack (or junk) foods. If they discovered their teenager was buying additional sweets or snacks, most of the middle class parents described challenging or reprimanding them. Others said they severely limited having biscuits or snacks in the house (Judith's mother: 'I tend, rather than put temptation in her way, I tend just not to do it, so none of us have it'). Controlling and moulding teenagers' eating practices at home, particularly if they were not as healthy as these middle class parents wished, was often described like a family project (Backett-Milburn *et al.* in press).

Already, then, we can see that there were some differences between the environments in which our two sets of teenagers lived and the ways in which their parents spoke about looking after everyday eating practices at home. Both sets of parents identified the increasing autonomy of teenagers as a threat to healthy eating practices, as was the ready availability and attractiveness of 'junk' foods. Both sets of parents said that they tried to provide a good diet at home, though exactly what this comprised varied and the middle class interviews suggested a greater belief in their ability to control and mould teenagers' tastes and choices than did those of the working class. However, parents' views are not stand alone entities. Although our studies showed that parents were in overall charge of food provisioning and eating practices at home, health-relevant behaviour is interactive and teenagers are also creating meanings and practices for themselves (Wills *et al.* 2008). Against this backdrop of parental accounts we now examine what the teenagers themselves said about their food and family practices at home and how they spoke about the negotiations surrounding these processes between themselves and their parents.

Teenagers' accounts of negotiating food and family practices at home

Food provision in the family home: teenager perspectives on tastes, preferences and parental control

In study 1 (w/c) the working class teenagers offered a somewhat different view about the extent to which they could choose what they ate at home than did their parents, most of whom seemed to feel that it was up to the teenager to decide. Parents, especially mothers, were reported by the working class teenagers as having a great deal of control over what was available for them to eat at home. Almost all of the working class teenagers said they were not usually asked what they wanted to eat and the main food provider was rarely described as consulting with other family members about meals that were prepared. Many, however, described having some autonomy over what they actually chose to eat and where they could eat this. Only a minority of the working class teenagers said that they had to ask their parents before taking or preparing any food or drink at home. Jodie was unusual in saying, for example: 'my mum disnae trust me. Even when I make a cup o' tea, it's like "watch that water!"'.

The working class teenagers reported sometimes being asked if there were particular foods they would like bought in the family shopping; those who were not asked said they often requested particular foods, or brands of foods. They did not, however, always receive the foods they asked for and this, they explained, was related to the price being prohibitive or a parent forgetting. Parents and grandparents were also described as exerting some control when young people came home from school for their lunch. In these situations, according to the teenagers, parents/grandparents usually provided the food on a daily basis without asking young people what they wanted. Overall, however, the working class teenagers' interviews indicated that, where they identified opportunities for choice around food and eating practices at home, they regularly seemed to negotiate with parents or simply got their own way. Compared with the middle class teenagers this appeared to result in a much greater amount of freedom about what they themselves could choose to eat.

In addition, about half the working class teenagers reported that they ate differently from their families by sometimes or often preparing food for themselves. These teenagers said they made themselves something to eat so they could more easily organise their social lives, without relying on parents and parent's own timetables. The foods prepared by these teenagers were, typically, sandwiches, instant-noodles and food that could be heated up (e.g. tinned food) (Wills *et al.* 2008). Such independence in domestic food preparation was seldom reported by the middle class teenagers.

Almost all of the working class teenagers also reported that parents had rules or expectations about the kinds and amounts of food they might eat in the home. These included: particular foods being restricted (usually fizzy drinks, sweets, crisps and biscuits but sometimes milk, yogurt or fruit juice); having to ask before taking a snack or drink (although fruit was said to be readily available); and not being allowed to eat a snack when a main meal was about to be served. Lorna was one of several working class teenagers who described trying to override her mother's rules, as the quotation below illustrates.

> Interviewer: So does she ever know that you have taken more than one [bar of chocolate]?
> Lorna: Mmh, she usually searches me. When I walked away, like this morning she searched my school bag 'cause I was in the cupboard and I shut my bag really fast 'cause I have a big bottle of juice... of course she opened my bag to see how many sweets and that I had taken (laughter).

In these socio-economically disadvantaged families many working class teenagers appeared to accept that some food rules were necessary to ensure that no one in the family ate more than their 'fair share' of food (often so that food lasted until the next shopping trip). About a quarter of teenagers in study 1 (w/c) reported that certain foods were not to be eaten because they had been bought for other family members (for example, full sugar drinks for parents; 'diet' yogurts for an older sister) (Wills *et al.* 2008).

Nevertheless, echoing their parents' accounts, the young teenagers in our working class study clearly expressed their likes and dislikes regarding food and described how they managed to negotiate the foods they preferred and avoid those they disliked. Many of them commented that their food preferences were dissimilar to parents or siblings and spoke of how they managed to avoid eating the foods that other family members liked (particularly vegetables). Nicole, for example, rarely ate her evening meal with her mother, partly because of their different schedules, but also because she did not like the food her mother ate:

> Interviewer: Do you have [your meal] on your own or with your Mum or ...?
> Nicole: On my own, 'cause she's never in, and all she ever eats is tatties (potatoes) and I canny (cannot) bear tatties every day
> Interviewer: What, just tatties on their own?
> Nicole: Tatties, turnip and cabbage, I've had it a couple of times but I like pasta.

Being aware of their own food preferences and tastes seemed to lead many of the working class teenagers to label themselves as fussy or greedy eaters. Only a minority reported that their tastes had changed as they got older, which meant they were now prepared to try a greater range of foods. Fruit and vegetables were frequently described as the subject of particular argument between parents and young teenagers. Even though most parents and teenagers reported that they were encouraged to eat vegetables and salad, very few working class teenagers said they were willing to eat these. For example, Neil said peas were the only vegetable he liked, but then went on to explain:

> Neil: 'If the food looks dodgy, I dinnae eat it... [Mum] tries to make me sometimes, if she's haeing [having] green beans or that. She'll put a couple on my plate'
> Interviewer: 'Do you eat them?'

Neil: 'Nah'
(Wills *et al.* 2008)

From their interviews, the middle class teenagers appeared to have very limited autonomy and choice in relation to family meals. Parents' control and shaping of young people's food choices and consumption can be seen particularly in decisions regarding meal preparation. The majority of parents preparing meals were described as deciding on the food without consulting young people or other family members, although young people said they could make occasional requests. Compared to the way that parents catered for their individual tastes, as reported by teenagers in study 1 (w/c), most of the middle class teenagers said they shared similar tastes to the rest of their family. Overall they only commented on one or two things that they did not like in relation to the other family members and some commented that meals would be a compromise, incorporating the food liked by all family members. In a few families members would eat the same general meal but within that there were some limited adaptations to accommodate tastes, for example providing a different protein dish for a vegetarian alongside shared vegetables and carbohydrates. In general, however, these middle class teenagers seemed to accept that families should eat the same meals together and also that family members would fit in with each others' tastes and preferences to make that possible.

Moreover, although middle class teenagers said it was often parents who made decisions about both the kinds of food and portions sizes they ate, the majority also reported that they were expected to finish most of their meals, even foods they disliked. It was only the occasional interviewee who said s/he might be allowed not to eat something s/he really disliked. Those who wanted to leave food that they disliked usually described having to reach some sort of agreement with their parents. For example, one boy mentioned making a deal with his parents to finish one food item in order not to eat another. For all, vegetables tended to be non-negotiable. Again, like their parents and unlike most of the working class sample, middle class teenagers appeared to accept that they should eat a greater variety of foods and become less fussy as they got older, as the following quotation illustrates:

> Callum: It probably wasn't as bad if I left things when I was younger because em, just kind of when you're younger it's, I'd say it's probably expected that you wouldn't like many things but I would still probably be expected to eat most of the stuff that I didn't like. (Backett-Milburn *et al.* in press)

Many of the middle class teenagers did report some autonomy in the area of choosing and helping themselves to snacks at home. However, again, their interviews revealed that this was against the backdrop of clearly defined parental expectations, which, by and large, they adhered to. Many seemed to view such rules or expectations as allowing them to control their own consumption both in quantity and choice. Most of the middle class teenagers said they were allowed to help themselves to fruit and drinks but had to ask permission for snacks like crisps, biscuits and chocolate; other items, such as fizzy juice, were described as special treats. For some, choice of snacks was not a real option as only 'healthy' options were available. For example, Fiona said she did not have to ask permission for snacks because they were all sensible snacks and Anna said she was allowed to help herself to snacks because she was both responsible in her choices and not going to 'gorge' herself. However, it appeared that this autonomy was indeed still being monitored as a few middle class teenagers reported that their parents intervened if they did over-indulge in snacking, for example:

> Gareth: No. I mean if, if I am getting like over the top like, I will have eaten like four bananas or something in a night they'll say you know, 'stop'. Or if I've, you know I've been drinking too much fizzy juice or something like that, they'll just say 'stop'.

> Shona: Like say I took um... a Kit-Kat or something, she (mother) would find out the next day and we'd sit down for about ten minutes and she'd be sitting questioning us, asking me like 'did I take it?', 'why did I take it?' 'why didn't I ask?'.

The middle class teenagers' accounts of eating at home revealed a considerable degree of parental regulation. However, sitting at the table sharing a family meal was not described as a curtailment of freedom by them, but rather as a social event, an opportunity to chat to other family members. Families who did not eat together were seen as not engaging in 'family time'. Middle class teenagers' reports that parents made only limited accommodation for tastes and preferences did not necessarily seem to be viewed in a negative light as many said that they had similar tastes to the rest of the family or that they liked the food that was provided. They described being encouraged to try new foods and to eat what they had been served. Here, though, their discussions about leaving food behind appeared to be less about food wastage and more about having a varied diet, eating foods because these were 'healthy' and developing more sophisticated tastes.

Conclusion

These two linked studies have raised some interesting similarities and contrasts between young teenagers' experiences of domestic food and eating practices in differing socio economic groupings. Interestingly, both sets of teenagers described how they felt they were provided with foods at home over which they had relatively little control, these were largely choices made by their parents, predominantly their mothers. Few teenagers in either study reported trying to bend parental food rules or change parental food provisioning practices to any great degree. However, the middle class interviewees portrayed themselves as generally approving of the family food provided and prepared by parents at home, whereas many of the working class teenagers regularly chose to prepare food for themselves, particularly when this facilitated their social lives or not having to eat the same foods as their parents. In some ways, therefore, the working class teenagers seemed to have greater autonomy over what and where they actually ate.

Parents in both studies spoke of the teenage years as heralding potential changes in their children's food choices and eating practices, most notably that teenagers would have a taste for and more opportunities to eat junk food (Wills *et al.* 2009). However, with regard to what happened at home, the working class and middle class parents appeared to react to this in different ways. By and large, the middle class teenager was expected to strictly limit his/her snack or junk food intake and this was monitored by the parents. In comparison, most of the working class parents, although not unconcerned, nevertheless felt there was little they could do to control these teenager tastes.

Our qualitative interviews, however, enabled us to understand these apparent class-based differences within the habitus, or cultures, of these families. Teenagers' domestic food practices need also to be seen in the light of wider socio-economic circumstances and perceived opportunities. It seemed that the working class parents, although expressing wishes for a healthy diet, placed such issues fairly well down their 'hierarchies of worries' about their teenagers' presents and futures. Other concerns about their teenagers' lives were simply more pressing for them. In contrast, against the backdrop of relatively secure and healthy environments and reasonably assured future prospects for their teenagers, middle class parents were better able to focus on moulding their eating practices and tastes. Against this backdrop of 'hierarchies of luxury and choice' (Backett-Milburn *et al.* in press) a focus on their teenagers' appropriate food and eating practices also appeared to be part of the process of making the future middle class adult.

Notes

1. Study 1 (w/c) Obesity and diet in early adolescence: A qualitative study of diet-related risk behaviours and beliefs in Scottish families resident in areas of deprivation, was funded by the Research Unit in Health, Behavior and Change, University of Edinburgh and NHS Health Scotland.
2. http://www.scotland.gov.uk/News/Releases/2006/10/17104536.

References

Backett-Milburn, K. and Harden, J., 2004. How children and their families construct and negotiate risk, safety and danger. *Childhood*, 11 (4), 429–447.

Backett-Milburn, K., Wills, W.J., Gregory, S., and Lawton, J., 2006. Making sense of eating, weight and risk in the early teenage years: views and concerns of parents in poorer socio-economic circumstances. *Social Science and Medicine*, 63 (3), 624–635.

Backett-Milburn, K., Wills, W., Roberts, M.L., and Lawton, J., 2008. *Parents' & teenagers' conceptions of diet, weight & health: Does class matter?* Final report to the ESRC, Res 00231504. Swindon: ESRC.

Backett-Milburn, K.C., Wills, W.J., Roberts, M.L., and Lawton, J., in press. Food, eating and taste: parents' perspectives on the making of the middle class teenager. *Social Science and Medicine*.

Ball, K. and Crawford, D., 2005. Socioeconomic status and weight change in adults: a review. *Social Science and Medicine*, 60 (9), 1987–2010.

Bradley, H., 1996. *Fractured identities: changing patterns of inequality*. Cambridge: Polity Press.

Bourdieu, P., 1984. *Distinction: a social critique of the judgement of taste*. London: Routledge and Kegan Paul.

Boyatzis, R.E., 1998. *Transforming qualitative information: thematic analysis and code development*. Thousand Oaks, CA: Sage.

Britten, N., Jones, R., Murphy, E., and Stacy, R., 1995. Qualitative research methods in general practice. *Family Practice*, 12 (1), 104–114.

Caplan, P., 1997. Approaches to the study of food, health and identity. *In*: P. Caplan, ed. *Food, health and identity*. London: Routledge.

Christensen, P. and James, A., eds., 2000. *Research with children: perspectives and practices*. London: Falmer Press.

Colls, R. and Evans, B., 2008. Embodying responsibility: children's health and supermarket initiatives. *Environment and Planning A*, 40 (3), 615–631.

Crossley, N., 2004. Fat is a sociological issue: obesity rates in late modern 'body conscious' societies. *Social Theory and Health*, 2, 222–253.

Cunningham, C., 2003. A fruitful direction for research in children's geography: fat chance? *Children's Geographies*, 1 (1), 125–127.

Devine, C., Jastran, M., Jabs, J., Wethington, E., Farell, T.J., and Bisogni, C.A., 2006. 'A lot of sacrifices': work-family spillover and the food choice coping strategies of low-wage employed parents. *Social Science and Medicine*, 63, 2591–2603.

Dietz, W., 2001. The obesity epidemic in young children. *British Medical Journal*, 322, 313–314.

Dixey, R., Sahota, P., Atwal, S., and Turner, A., 2001. 'Ha ha, you're fat, we're strong'; a qualitative study of boys' and girls' perceptions of fatness, thinness, social pressures and health using focus groups. *Health Education*, 101 (5), 206–216.

D'Houtard, A. and Field, M., 1984. Images of health: variations in perceptions by social class in a French population. *Sociology of Health and Illness*, 6, 30–60.

Dowler, E. and Calvert, C., 1995. Looking for 'fresh' food: diet and lone parents. *Proceedings of the Nutrition Society*, 54, 759–769.

Dowling, R., 2009. Geographies of identity: landscapes of class. *Progress in Human Geography*, 33, 833–839.

Eckert, G., 2004. 'If I tell them then I can': ways of relating to adult rules. *Childhood*, 11 (1), 9–26.

Egger, G. and Swinburn, B., 1997. An 'ecological' approach to the obesity pandemic. *British Medical Journal*, 315, 477–480.

Eldridge, J. and Murcott, A., 2000. Adolescents' dietary habits and attitudes: unpacking the 'problem' of (parental) influence. *Health*, 4 (1), 25–49.

Grieshaber, S., 1997. Mealtime rituals: power and resistance in the construction of mealtime rules. *British Journal of Sociology*, 48 (4), 649–666.

Kaufman, L. and Karpati, A., 2007. Understanding the sociocultural roots of childhood obesity: food practices among Latino families of Bushwick, Brooklyn. *Social Science and Medicine*, 64, 2177–2188.

Lupton, D., 1994. Food, memory and meaning: the symbolic and social nature of food events. *The Sociological Review*, 42 (4), 686–702.

Metcalfe, A., Owen, J., Shipton, G., and Dryden, C., 2008. Inside and outside the school lunchbox: themes and reflections. *Children's Geographies*, 6 (4), 403–412.

Morgan, D., 1996. *Family connections*. Cambridge: Polity.

Pike, J., 2008. Foucault, space and primary school dining rooms. *Children's Geographies*, 6 (4), 413–422.

Reay, D., 2005. Beyond consciousness? The psychic landscape of social class. *Sociology*, 39 (5), 911–928.

Sarlio-Lahteenkorva, S., 2007. Determinants of long-term weight maintenance. *Acta Paediatrica*, 96, 26–28.

Seaman, P., Turner, K., Hill, M., Walker, M., and Stafford, A., 2006. *Parenting and children's resilience in disadvantaged communities*. London: National Children's Bureau.

Shaw, A., McMunn, A., and Field, J., 2000. *The Scottish health survey 1998*. London: Joint Health Surveys Unit.

Sproston, K. and Primatesta, P., 2003. *Health survey for England 2003: risk factors for cardiovascular disease*. London: The Stationery Office.

Tomanovic, S., 2004. Family habitus as the cultural context for childhood. *Childhood*, 11, 339–360.

Valentine, G., 1999. Eating in: home, consumption and identity. *The Sociological Review*, 47 (3), 491–524.

Warin, M., Turner, K., Moore, V., and Davies, M., 2008. Bodies, mothers and identities: rethinking obesity and the BMI. *Sociology of Health and Illness*, 30 (1), 97–111.

West, P. and Sweeting, H., 2004. Evidence on equalisation in health in youth from the West of Scotland. *Social Science and Medicine*, 59, 13–27.

Wills, W.J., Backett-Milburn, K., Gregory, S., and Lawton, J., 2008. 'If the food looks dodgy I dinnae eat it': teenagers' accounts of food and eating practices in socio-economically disadvantaged families. *Sociological Research Online*, 13 (1).

Wills, W.J., Backett-Milburn, K., Lawton, J., and Roberts, E.M., 2009. Consuming fast food: the perceptions and practices of middle class young teenagers. *In*: A. James, V. Tingstad and A. Kjørholt, eds. *Children, food and identity in everyday life*. London: Palgrave.

Williams, S., 1995. Theorising class, health and lifestyles: can Bourdieau help us? *Sociology of Health and Illness*, 17 (5), 577–604.

Williams, S.J., 2003. *Medicine and the body*. London: Sage.

Wright-St Clair, V., Hocking, C., Bunrayong, W., Vittayakorn, S., and Rattakorn, P., 2005. Older New Zealand women doing the work of Christmas: a recipe for identity formation. *The Sociological Review*, 53 (2), 332–350,

Discussant piece: how parenting education and family learning can be set within a tiered intervention framework to aid the development of healthy eating practices

Catriona Rioch
Team Leader, Early Years Resource Team, Perth & Kinross Council, Perth, UK

Whilst there are similarities in themes emerging from the two studies by Curtis *et al.* (this issue) and Backett-Milburn *et al.* (this issue), there are some differences. Curtis *et al.*'s (this issue) study seems to imply that children and parents, across a range of geographical areas and differing demographic profiles, have a degree of shared understanding about what constitutes unhealthy eating. Also the symbolic importance of 'eating together' as a family has not lost its potency. However, Backett-Milburn *et al.*'s (this issue) study implies that whilst middle class families share similar views and understanding as those in the Curtis *et al.* (this issue) study, there is a distinction. Parents from working class backgrounds have less understanding or focus on healthy eating and allow much more autonomy around their children's eating habits. There is a major difference between socio-economic classes in terms of the amount of control parents feel they should or could exercise over their teenagers' consumption of food.

Curtis *et al.*'s (this issue) study explicitly draws out conclusions about eating practices as affecting and affected by the parent–child relationship and influencing and being influenced by family values. This theme is touched on also, in Beckett-Milburn *et al.*'s (this issue) study where middle class families more consciously link eating together as 'family time'. In working class families eating habits were not viewed as unimportant, simply as less important, and these families seem to be less conscious of any link to the impact these habits might have on the quality of family life and relationships.

Whilst there are these differences between the work of Curtis *et al.* (this issue) and Backett-Milburn *et al.* (this issue), there are two overarching themes which emerge:

- Parenting styles
- Parental understanding of child development

Parenting styles

The way in which parenting styles affect how parents regulate or do not regulate their children's eating habits.

Child development

> The way in which parental understanding about how parents should help children and young people achieve maturational tasks, appropriate to their stage of development, appears to influence how they regulate or do not regulate their children's eating habits.

It would appear that a focus on supporting parenting and family learning must be a central component to any policy or practice development in improving the eating habits of families at all ages. The Change 4 Life programme cite research,[1] that the risk of obesity amongst children age 4–5 is significantly greater among parents classified as 'permissive' – indulgent, 'neglectful' – emotionally uninvolved and particularly 'authoritarian' compared to 'authoritative' parents (Rhee *et al.* 2006). How then can we help more parents achieve an authoritative style?

In Scotland some local authorities have developed parenting strategies which are built on a tiered intervention framework (levels of need and targeting) and linked to an Integrated Assessment Framework. Perhaps a focus on healthy eating could be integrated more into this? Can we have more accessible, evidence based practice and research about healthy eating – what works for whom and at what age and level of need?

Similar to the parents in Backett-Milburn *et al.*'s (this issue) study, eating practices for many professionals can be low in the 'hierarchy of worries' about children. In my experience services specifically addressing healthy eating are often considered as an 'add on' or specialised service, separate from other main stream or targeted services. Within the latter, healthy eating may not be addressed at all unless the problems are so significant that eating practices are assessed as a part of chronic neglect.

How can we integrate an approach to healthy eating into ALL services and all aspects of our work no matter what level of need we are addressing? If we set out levels of need of families within a common tiered intervention framework, a staged, integrated and more dynamic approach could perhaps be used to encourage healthy eating practices. Much work often needs to be undertaken to address parents' own needs, raise their self esteem and confidence before they can access local and/or universal services.

As practitioners we should be much more conscious that by addressing parenting skills, promoting attachment, helping parents understand the stage of their children's development better, we are in fact setting a base line to aid improvement of healthy eating practices. We should also do more to explicitly link parenting, attachment and eating practices and raise awareness about how interdependent these areas are. Should parenting programmes include a module around eating and explicit links between parenting styles and eating practices?

Early intervention

We should also be mindful about early intervention, although there will always be a need for targeted services, prevention is better than cure. In the service I am currently managing it is clear that there is a lack of understanding about the timing and process of weaning for both parents and grandparents. Many do not understand the implications of using too much convenience food, salt/sugar content in foods or even when to start weaning. Although they may receive advice verbally from health or other professionals, rarely are they actually shown how and what to cook. (Our service is developing a 'weaning pack' for parents.)

We have an opportunity through the Scottish Government's (Scottish Government 2009)[2] new Early Years Framework, to invest more in the Early Years. Ideally, wherever possible, action on improving healthy eating should begin in the early years – starting at the ante natal stage with pregnant women.

Priorities of the Early Years Framework include:

- Developing a coherent approach – local partners will start the process of aligning local resources to local priorities for action.
- Breaking the cycle of poverty, inequality and poor outcomes in and through early years.
- Simplifying and streamlining delivery – provide a more coordinated set of supports for children and families, building on integrated services planning.

All of these can and should include specific approaches to improving eating practices within families in Scotland. The work in this volume by Curtis *et al.* (this issue) and Backett-Milburn *et al.* (this issue) indicate that parenting styles and parental understanding of child development influence children's eating habits. In order to improve eating practices of families, parenting and family learning should be a central component in policy and practice development. There is an opportunity, through the Scottish Government's Early Years Framework, to ensure a focus on healthy eating practices is set within a tiered level of service provision from universal to targeted.

Notes

1. COI for Department of Health and the Department for Children, Schools and Families. 2008, *Change 4 life*. Crown copyright November.
2. Early Years Framework, Scottish Government. 2009. ISBN 9780755959426 www.scotland.gov.uk/publications/2009.

Reference

Rhee, K.E., Lumeng, J.C., and Appugliese, D.P., 2006. Parenting styles and overweight status in first grade. *Pediatrics*, 117 (6), 2047–2054.

Index

Abrams, L. 24
Aitken, S. 2
Alanen, L. 74
Alcock, S. 1
Alderson, P.: and Morrow, M. 22
Allan, G.: and Crow, G. 23
Amin, Idi 15
Anglin, J. 24
Arias, S.: and Warf, B. 2
asylum-seeking children 7–14
Ayotte, W. 12

Backett-Milburn, K.: *et al* 3–4, 67, 77–91;
   and Harden, J. 79
Ball, K.: and Crawford, D. 78
Balls, Ed 43
Barker, J.: and Smith, F. 50, 52
Bell, D.: and Valentine, G. 66
Blair, Tony 42
Blake, M.: *et al* 66
Blears, Hazel 42
Blishen, E. 47
Blunt, A. 22; and Dowling, R. 23
Bordieu, P. 78–9
Boyatzis, R. 80
Bradley, H. 78
Brembeck, H. 67
Brindley, M. 42
British Association for Adoption and
   Fostering 14
Britten, N.: *et al* 79
Burke, C.: and Grosvenor, I. 39, 46–7
Buttriss, J. 51

Calvert, C.: and Dowler, E. 79
Caplan, P. 78
Caroline Walker Trust 42
Catling, S. 50
Centre for Research on Families and
   Relationships (CRFR) 2
Charles, N.: and Kerr, M. 66
Charon, J. 1
Chase, E.: *et al* 10–11

Child Poverty Action Group 42
child-centred service provision 25
Children Act (1989) 8
Children as Family Participants study 68–74
Children and Young People Unit 42
Children's Geographies journal 2
Choosing a Better Diet (DoH) 41
Choosing Health (DoH) 41
Christensen, P.: *et al* 2, 27, 73; and James, A.
   40, 46, 79
Coleman, T.: and Collins, D. 50
Colls, R.: and Evans, B. 78
Colquhoun, D.: *et al* 52
Connolly, H.: Kohli, R. and Warman, A. 3–
   5, 7–19, 35–8
Cook, D. 69, 74
Coveney, J. 73
Crawford, D.: and Ball, K. 78; and Jeffrey, R.
   67
Crossley, N. 78
Crow, G.: and Allan, G. 23
Cunningham, C. 1–2, 63, 78
Curtis, P.: *et al* 3–5, 66, 75, 89–91; James, A.
   and Ellis, K. 65–76

Daily Mail 54, 65
Daniel, P.: and Gustafsson, U. 3–4, 39–48,
   63–4
Department for Education and Science
   (DfES) 40–1; *Working Together* 40
Department for the Environment, Food and
   Rural Affairs (DEFRA) 41
Department of Health (DoH) 41; *Choosing a
   Better Diet* 41; *Choosing Health* 41
Dequech, D. 28
Devault, M. 66, 77
Devine, C.: *et al* 78
d'Houtard, A.: and Field, M. 78
Dickie, J. 63
Dietz, W. 77
Dixey, R.: *et al* 77–8
Dockar-Drysdale, B. 37
Dorrer, N.: *et al* 3–5, 21–33, 35–7

Douglas, M. 24
Dowler, E.: and Calvert, C. 79
Dowling, R. 78; and Blunt, A. 23
Du Bois, C.: and Mintz, S. 8

Early Years Framework 90–1
Eastmond, M. 11
Eckert, G. 79
Economic and Social Research Council
   (ESRC) 2
Education (Provision of Meals) Act (1906) 50
Education School Meals and Nutrition Bill
   (2005) 51
Egger, G.: and Swinburn, B. 78
Eldridge, J.: and Murcott, A. 79, 81
Ellis, K.: Curtis, P. and James, A. 65–76
Emond, R. 1–6, 22; McIntosh, I. and Punch,
   S. 63–4
Evans, B.: and Colls, R. 78

Faiges-Hijon, A. 10
Field, M.: and d'Houtard, A. 78
Fielding, S. 50
Finch, J. 31
Fischler, C. 47
food and food practices 1–6, 63–4; first refuge
   12–13; meanings and success measurement
   4–5; security and survival 9–10, 13–14;
   space and contexts 2–4
Food in Schools Programme 41–2
Food Standards Agency (FSA) 41; *Shaping
   the eating habits of the next generation* 42
foster care 11–17
Foster Care Associates 14
Foucault, M. 50, 52–3
Fredmann, S.: and Morris, G. 53

Gagen, E. 50
Gallagher, M. 53, 57
Giddens, A. 28
Gillis, J. 67
Goffman, E. 24, 28
Green, T.: *et al* 67
Grieshaber, S. 1, 79
Grosvenor, I.: and Burke, C. 39, 46–7
Gustafsson, U. 50–1; and Daniel, P. 3–4, 39–
   48

Harden, J.: and Backett-Milburn, K. 79
Harrell-Bond, B.: *et al* 9
Harris, G.: and Passmore, S. 50
Health and Safety regulations 29
Healthy Eating initiative 39–43
healthy eating practices 89–91; child
   development 90–1; parenting styles 89
Healthy Living Blueprint for schools 41

Hearing Experiences of Asylum and
   Resettlement (HEAR ME) study 11–16
Hepworth, M. 23
Herbert, J. 8
Higgins, J. 30
Hill, M.: and Hopkins, P. 12
Hofman, C.: *et al* 9
Holloway, S.: and Valentine, G. 2, 50
Holt, L. 57–8
Home Office 8
Hopkins, P.: and Hill, M. 12

institutional control 29
Integrated Assessment Framework 90

Jackson, P. 1, 67; *et al* 66
James, A.: and Christensen, P. 40, 46, 79;
   Curtis, P. and Ellis, K. 65–76; *et al* 1–2, 23,
   50, 55, 66–7
Jeffery, R.: and Crawford, D. 67
Johansson, B.: *et al* 70

Karpati, A.: and Kaufman, L. 78
Kearns, R.: *et al* 49
Keith, M.: and Pile, S. 2
Kerr, M.: and Charles, N. 66
Kershner, R. 50
Kime, N. 63
Kohli, R.: Connolly, H. and Warman, A. 3–
   5, 7–19, 35–8

Lawler, S. 56
Lawton, J.: *et al* 77–88
Lemke, T. 53
Lipsett, A. 43, 47
London Local Authority (LA) 43
Löw, M. 2, 28
Lupton, D. 66, 77

McIntosh, I. 1–6; *et al* 31; Punch, S. and
   Emond, R. 63–4
McKendrick, J. 1–2, 63–4
McRae, J.: and Zwi, A. 9
Madigan, R.: and Munro, M. 23
Maguire, M. 54, 56
Malone, K.: and Tranter, P. 50
Marte, L. 8
Mayall, B. 47, 55–6
Metcalfe, A.: *et al* 1, 79
Mintz, S.: and Du Bois, C. 8, 78
Mohr, J.: and White, H. 28
Montgomery, E.: and Von Folsach, L. 10
moralities and family life 65–76; *Children as
   Family Participants* study 68–74; other
   food practices 68–71; snacking 65–71, 74
Morgan, D. 66–7, 75, 77
Morgan, K. 51

Morris, G.: and Fredmann, S. 53
Morrow, V. 52; and Alderson, P. 22
Moss, P.: and Petrie, P. 28, 32, 35, 39–43, 47
Munro, M.: and Madigan, R. 23
Murcott, A. 66; and Eldridge, J. 79, 81
Murphy, E. 72–3

National Fruit and Vegetable Scheme 41
National Health Service (NHS) 65; Change 4
  Life campaign 65, 71, 90
National Healthy Schools Programme 41
Nelson, M.: and Paul, A. 55

Office of National Statistics (NS-SEC) 80;
  Family Affluence Scale 80
Oliver, Jamie 51, 72

Parsons, E.: et al 49
Passmore, S.: and Harris, G. 50
Paul, A.: and Nelson, M. 55
Personal, Social, Health and Citizenship
  Education (PSHCE) 54
Pervasive Refusal Syndrome 10
Petrie, P.: and Moss, P. 28, 32, 35, 39–43, 47
Pike, J. 1–5, 40–2, 47, 49–61, 63, 79
Pile, S.: and Keith, M. 2
Pooley, C.: et al 49
Primatesta, P.: and Sproston, K. 67, 79
Prout, A. 70
psychological perspectives 35–8
Punch, S. 1–6, 52; et al 22; McIntosh, I. and
  Emond, R. 63–4

Reay, D. 54, 79
Recipes for Fostering initiative 14–17; carers
  and 'The Review Cake' 16–17
residential child care 21–38; children's
  experiences 26–8; Corporate Parents 36;
  home as an institution and workplace 28–
  31; staff strategies 24–6; study and
  objectives 22–31, 22; workers 36
resistance strategies 3
Rethinking Residential Child Care (Smith) 35
Rhee, K.: et al 90
Rioch, C. 89–91
Roberts, M-L.: et al 77–88
Robinson, V.: and Segrott, J. 10

Sarlio-Lahteenkorva, S. 78
Scheper-Hughes, N. 13, 38
School Food Trust 43, 51
school lunches 39–48; eating and playing 45–
  6; getting served 44–5; policies 41–3;
  power, discipline and resistance 5, 49–61;
  study 43–6, 51–9; supervision responsibility
  53–6
School Meals Review Panel 42

School Meals Service 50–1; history 50–1
Scott, R. 28
Scottish Index of Deprivation 80
Segrott, J.: and Robinson, V. 10
Sellen, D.: et al 10
Sen, A. 9
Seymour, J. 2, 21
Shaping the eating habits of the next
  generation (FSA) 42
Shaw, A.: et al 67, 79
Shoham, J. 9
Short, J. 23
Silva, E.: and Smart, C. 21, 66
Simic, C. 10
Sinclair, I. 8
Skeggs, B. 54
Smart, C. 69; and Silva, E. 21, 66
Smith, F.: and Barker, J. 50, 52
Smith, M. 24; Rethinking Residential Child
  Care 35
Social Services Departments 8
spatiality 2–3
Sproston, K.: and Primatesta, P. 67, 79
Stanley, J. 35–8
Stanley, K. 10
Stern, D. 37
Summerfield, D. 9
Sweeting, H.: and West, P. 79
Swinburn, B.: and Egger, G. 78

teenagers and their food practices 77–88; does
  class matter? 78–86; parental perspectives
  80–3
Thompson, S. 50
Tomanovic, S. 79
Tranter, P.: and Malone, K. 50
Turton, D. 9

United Nations (UN) 7–8; Convention on the
  Rights of the Child (UNCRC) 7–8, 11, 17;
  High Commission for Refugees (UNHCR)
  7–9
University Research Ethics 68

Valentine, G. 2, 40, 49, 55, 77; and Bell, D.
  66; and Holloway, S. 2, 50
Vanderbeck, R. 32
Von Folsach, L.: and Montgomery, E. 10

Wade, J.: et al 10
Walters, S. 54
Warf, B.: and Arias, S. 2
Warin, M.: et al 78–9
Warman, A.: Kohli, R. and Connolly, H. 7–
  19, 35–8
Welshman, J. 50
West, C.: and Zimmerman, D. 21

West, P.: and Sweeting, H. 79
White, H.: and Mohr, J. 28
Willets, A. 66
Williams, S. 78
Willcocks, D.: *et al* 28
Wills, W.: *et al* 2, 77–88
Winnicott, D. 35–7
Winterman, D. 42
Women of Rawmarsh 51

Working Together (DfES) 40
Wright-St Clair, V.: *et al* 77–8

Zieher, H. 67
Zimmerman, D.: and West, C. 21
Zwi, A.: and McRae, J. 9

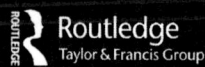
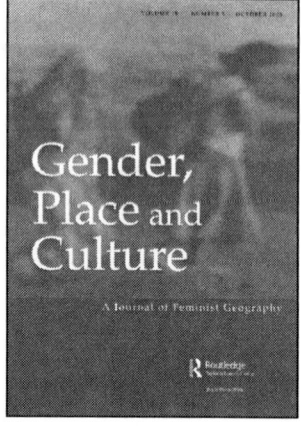
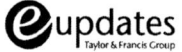
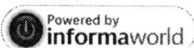
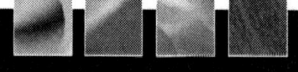

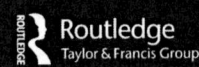

Annals of the Association of American Geographers

Published on behalf of the Association of American Geographers

CELEBRATING ITS CENTENARY ISSUE IN 2010!

EDITORS:
Mark Fonstad, *Texas State University, USA*
Audrey Kobayashi, *Queen's University, USA*
Mei-Po Kwan, *The Ohio State University, USA*
Karl Zimmerer, *The Pennsylvania State University, USA*

As the flagship journal of the Association of American Geographers, ***Annals of the Association of American Geographers*** publishes original, timely, and innovative peer-reviewed articles that advance knowledge in all facets of the discipline. These articles address significant research problems and issues, and are attuned to the sensibilities of a diverse scholarly audience. In addition to articles in four major areas - Environmental Sciences; Methods, Models, and Geographic Information Sciences; Nature and Society; and People, Place, and Region - the ***Annals*** publishes integrative and cross-cutting papers, commentaries, review articles, forums, book reviews, and occasional map supplements.

To view free articles please visit **www.tandf.co.uk/journals/aag** and click on News & Offers.

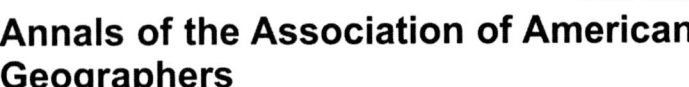

Annals
of the Association
of American Geographers

2008 Impact Factor 2.679, Ranked 6/51 (Geography)

©2009 Thomson Reuters, Journal Citation Reports®

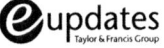
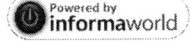

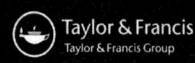
Taylor & Francis
Taylor & Francis Group

The Professional Geographer

Forum and Journal of the Association of American Geographers

EDITOR:
Sharmistha Bagchi-Sen, *State University of New York, USA*

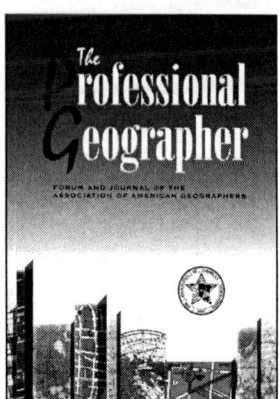

Addressing questions and problems of interest to a wide group of geographers, *The Professional Geographer,* published for the Association of American Geographers provides a forum for new ideas and alternative viewpoints in academic and applied geography. The journal publishes concise research articles ranging in content and approach from the rigorously analytic to the broadly philosophical. It also includes brief reviews of important new publications, as well as occasional focus sections and discussions of topics of particular interest.

To view free articles please visit **www.tandf.co.uk/journals/pg** and click on News & Offers.

To sign up for tables of contents, new publications and citation alerting services visit www.informaworld.com/alerting

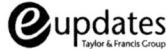
updates
Taylor & Francis Group

Register your email address at **www.tandf.co.uk/journals/eupdates.asp** to receive information on books, journals and other news within your areas of interest.

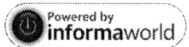
Powered by
informaworld

For further information, please contact Customer Services at either of the following:
T&F Informa UK Ltd, Sheepen Place, Colchester, Essex, CO3 3LP, UK
Tel: +44 (0) 20 7017 5544 Fax: 44 (0) 20 7017 5198
Email: subscriptions@tandf.co.uk

Taylor & Francis Inc, 325 Chestnut Street, Philadelphia, PA 19106, USA
Tel: +1 800 354 1420 (toll-free calls from within the US)
or +1 215 625 8900 (calls from overseas) Fax: +1 215 625 2940
Email: customerservice@taylorandfrancis.com

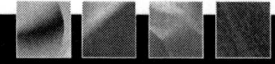

View an online sample issue at:
www.tandf.co.uk/journals/pg